Advanced Drug Delivery Systems

Edited by Bhupendra Prajapati

Published in London, United Kingdom

Advanced Drug Delivery Systems
http://dx.doi.org/10.5772/intechopen.100967
Edited by Bhupendra Prajapati

Contributors
Bhupendra Gopalbhai Prajapati, Kapil Gore, Sankha Bhattacharya, Vishal Pande, Ajinkya Pote, Vikas Ahirrao, Anjali Prashant Bedse, Deepa Singh, Shilpa Raut, Aarti Wable, Samiksha Pagar, Prajwal Pagare, Samruddha Wavikar, Kajal Baviskar, Luz Eugenia Eugenia Alcántara-Quintana, Carlos Miguel Lopez-Mendoza, Ana Jared Tenorio-Salazar, Amal H. El-Kamel, Asmaa A. Ashour, Vikas Pandey, Tanweer Haider, Poornima Agrawal, Sakshi Soni, Vandana Soni, Paul Rodriques

First published in London, United Kingdom, 2023 by IntechOpen
IntechOpen is the global imprint of INTECHOPEN LIMITED, registered in England and Wales, registration number: 11086078, 5 Princes Gate Court, London, SW7 2QJ, United Kingdom

British Library Cataloguing-in-Publication Data
A catalogue record for this book is available from the British Library

Additional hard and PDF copies can be obtained from orders@intechopen.com

Advanced Drug Delivery Systems
Edited by Bhupendra Prajapati
p. cm.
Print ISBN 978-1-80356-983-3
Online ISBN 978-1-80356-984-0
eBook (PDF) ISBN 978-1-80356-985-7

Meet the editor

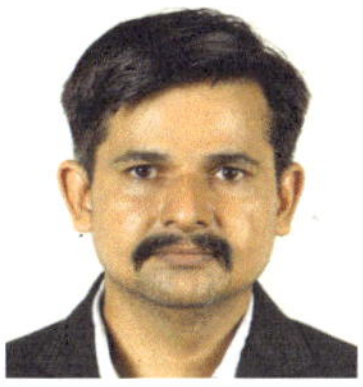

Dr. Bhupendra Prajapati is a professor in the Faculty of Pharmacy, at Ganpat University, India. He has more than 20 years of academic and research experience. He has published more than 100 research and review papers in international and national journals. He has also edited eight books and authored twenty-five book chapters. He is the recipient of various awards, recognitions, and grants from national and international authorities. He has three Indian patents to his credit and three applications under evaluation. Dr. Prajapati is a reviewer for three high-impact journals and is on the editorial board of several others. He is an active life member of IPA, APTI, and CRSIC. His current research focus is a lipid-based drug delivery and nanotech formulations.

Contents

Preface

This book describes important information about drug delivery systems used for the treatment of various diseases. These systems improve the therapeutic effect of drugs either by targeting or delivering drugs at a specific rate to the desired site. The content of this book is useful for undergraduates and postgraduate students in sciences, pharmacy, and medicine as well as researchers and professionals familiar with the principles of drug delivery systems. The book focuses on unique drug delivery systems, strategy, technology, formulation-based approaches, and tailored systems established for the safe administration and within-body transportation of pharmaceuticals as needed for the greatest therapeutic advantages with the least amount of side effects possible. The introductory chapter on advanced drug delivery systems discusses conventional vs advanced drug delivery benefits. It also covers the various carrier systems used and approaches used in the last few decades.

Chapter 2, "Advances in Natural Polymeric Nanoparticles for the Drug Delivery", describes the key advantages of natural and biodegradable polymers in the development of various drug delivery systems. The complexity of diseases and the intrinsic drug toxicity and side effects have led to an interest in the development and optimization of drug delivery systems. The advancements in nanotechnology have favored the development of novel formulations that can modulate the biopharmaceutical properties of bioactives and thus improve their pharmacological and therapeutic action. The shape, size, and charge of nanoscale delivery systems, such as nanoparticles (NPs), are required to be investigated and changed to promote and optimize formulations. The various natural polymeric NPs (PNPs) are key for enhancing bioavailability or specific delivery to a certain site of action. This chapter describes the uses of various polymeric materials for the development of NPs as drug-delivery systems for various ailments. The entrapment of bioactive compounds in PNP systems is a hopeful move toward the improvement of the efficacy of drugs in the treatment of various diseases.

Chapter 3, "Recent Strategies for Ocular Drug Delivery: Promises and Challenges", discusses various systems to target the anterior and posterior segments of the eye. The unique anatomy and physiology of the eye lead to challenges in efficient ocular drug delivery. Nanoscience is emerging as an important tool in the development of novel strategies for ocular disease management. Various active molecules have been designed to associate with nanocarriers to overcome ocular barriers and interact with certain ocular tissues. This chapter examines barriers to intraocular delivery, general pathways for ocular absorption, and factors affecting intraocular bioavailability. It provides insight into such systems as nanomicelles, nanoparticles, nanosuspensions, vesicular systems, in situ gel, dendrimers, contact lenses, implants, microneedles, and cell-based delivery systems as well as gene-based ocular delivery systems.

Chapter 4, "Recent Pharmaceutical Developments in the Treatment of Cancer Using Nanosponges", discusses nanosponges, a class of nanoparticles characterized by their sponge-like surface that ensures high loading capacity in the treatment of cancer. The chapter discusses nanosponges and their synthesis, characterization, optimization, and applications in cancer. According to the literature, nanosponges can be classified based on their starting materials, which could be polymers, metals, or metal oxides, among other materials. Polymer nanosponges can be manufactured by methods such as the melt method, emulsion method, solvent method, and ultrasound-assisted method. Metallic nanosponges are manufactured by methods such as dealloying and sol–gel methods. Factors related to drugs or process parameters influence the formation of nanosponges. These process parameters have been used by many researchers to optimize the formulation of nanosponges to achieve optimum results related to loading efficiency, particle size, and encapsulation efficiency. Polymer structure also affects the formation of nanosponges. The chapter concludes with examples of using nanosponges for the delivery of anticancer drugs and current research trends.

Chapter 5, "Organogel: A Propitious Carman in Drug Delivery System", discusses the types, properties, synthesis/manufacturing, and applications of organogel. Types of organogels include lecithin organogels, pluronic lecithin organogels, limonene GP1/PG organogels, micro-emulsion based organogels (MBG) stabilized by gelatin, sorbitan organogels derived from fatty acids, polyethylene organogels, eudragit organogels, supramolecular organogels, and L-alanine-derived organogels. The chapter highlights the limitations of organogels as drug delivery systems. It describes various properties of organogels, including viscoelasticity, thermostability, thermoreversibility, non-birefringence, optical clarity, chirality effect, and biocompatibility. It also discusses the role of different organogelators like aryl cyclohexanol derivatives, polymer organogels, gemini organogelator, Boc-Ala(1)-Aib(2)-β-Ala(3)-OMe organogelators, and low-molecular weight organogelators (LMWOs) in formulating organogels. The chapter presents methods for the preparation of organogels such as the fluid-filled fiber method, solid fiber method, hydration method, and other novel methods. The chapter also explains factors affecting organogels, such as pH, temperature, moisture, type of organogelators, and moisture. Finally, it gives detailed applications of organogels in oral, topical, parenteral, and ocular drug delivery systems with suitable examples.

Chapter 6, "Transdermal Delivery of Drugs for Acute and Chronic Pain", discusses the application of transdermal drug delivery systems (TDDS) for the effective management of pain. The chapter explains the historical development of transdermal systems, key advantages and limitations, formulation composition/approaches, typical properties, and application of TDDS as carriers for drugs. It concludes that there are several patch options available on the market for the treatment of acute and chronic pain. TDDS is an attractive option because of its advantages over other systems (pills, tablets). It promotes pharmaceutical adhesion because it is a non-invasive method of dosage and self-administration. However, considerations must be made in diminishing the secondary and adverse effects of current TDDS and in combining new nanosystems for drug encapsulation for better control of the release. In future outlooks, new smart TDDS are being developed that include external stimuli for the release of the drug.

Chapter 7, "Mesoporous Silica Based Cancer Theranostic: A Modern Approach in Upcoming Medicine", explains the utilization of mesoporous silica micro/nanoparticles to load therapeutic and diagnostic agents for targeting cancer. The chapter discusses major challenges in targeting and treating cancer along with various diagnosis methods. It provides detailed information about nanoparticles as targeted drug delivery systems with special emphasis on mesoporous silica nanoparticles and their formulation, properties, biocompatibility, biodegradability, toxicity, and safety.

Bhupendra Prajapati
Shree S.K.Patel College of Pharmaceutical Education and Research,
Ganpat University,
Mahesana, India

Chapter 1

Introductory Chapter: Advanced Drug Delivery Systems

Sankha Bhattacharya, Paul Rodriques and Bhupendra Prajapati

1. Introduction

"The process or method of providing a pharmaceutical substance to have a therapeutic effect in people or animals is known as drug delivery" [1]. A drug's compliance, safety, and efficacy can all be greatly enhanced by transforming it from its traditional form into a unique delivery system. An old drug molecule can be given new life with the use of an advance drug delivery system (ADDS). Various technological advances of unit operations such as drying, filtration, and mixing also help to advancement in modification and improvement in formulations [2]. With the right design, an ADDS can be a game-changer for addressing issues connected with targeted drug delivery. Pharmaceutical companies have been working on innovative drug delivery systems due to the growing demand for safer, more effective methods of administering drugs to patients.

The form in which a drug is administered can have a substantial impact on its efficacy. Some molecules have a range of optimal doses where the greatest benefit is obtained; dosages outside or inside of this range may be hazardous or have no therapeutic value at all [3]. The very gradual improvement in the effectiveness of treating serious diseases, on the other hand, has indicated an increasing need for a multidisciplinary approach to the delivery of medicines to target tissues. As a result, advanced methods for modifying pharmacological effects such as pharmacokinetics, pharmacodynamics, nonspecific toxicity, immunogenicity, biorecognition, and efficacy have been developed [4, 5]. Polymer science, pharmaceutics, bioconjugate chemistry, and molecular biology have all come together to form these advance techniques, which are collectively known as drug delivery systems [6, 7]. Various drug delivery and drug targeting approaches are being developed to limit drug breakdown and loss, reduce undesired side effects, enhance drug bioavailability and the proportion of drugs deposited in the appropriate location. What was once a fantasy or dream, controlled and advance drug delivery is now a reality. Over the past 15 years, researchers from pharmaceutical companies and other institutions have conducted exhaustive studies in this area of drug development. There are many different types of drug carriers, including soluble polymers, insoluble or biodegradable microparticles, natural and synthetic polymers, microcapsules, lipoproteins, liposomes, and micelles [7–10]. The carriers can be designed to break down slowly, respond to stimuli (such as pH or temperature), and be selectively delivered to their intended target (e.g., by conjugating them with specific antibodies against certain characteristic components of the area of interest). In order to deliver the drug to where it needs to go, you need to be able to "target" it. Two main approaches of targeting the sites of drug release: I. Non-active methods;

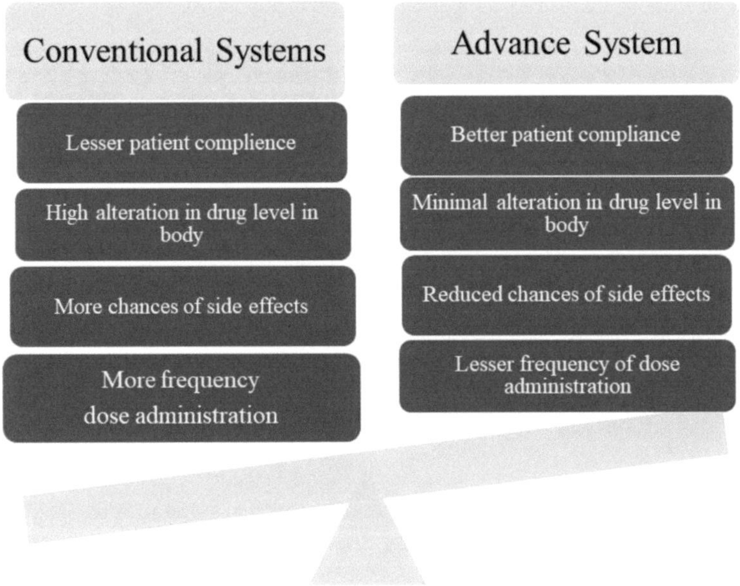

Figure 1.
Convectional vs ADDS.

II. Directed methods. The increased vascular permeability of tumor tissues relative to healthy tissue results in the preferential accumulation of chemotherapeutic drugs in solid tumors, an example of passive targeting. Surface functionalization of drug carriers with ligands that are selectively recognized by receptors on the surface of the cells of interest is a strategy that could enable active targeting. Given the selectivity of ligand-receptor interactions, this could lead to more targeted drug delivery. One definition of a drug delivery system is a system that consists of two components: (a) a drug formulation, and (b) a medical device or dosage form/technology designed to deliver the medication to its intended site of action inside the body. It has been discovered that certain dosage forms have significant drawbacks, such as increased toxicity, decreased efficiency, and unpleasant side effects. As the healthcare industry has grown, new drug delivery systems have been developed or are in the works to address the shortcomings of the existing drug administration methods. Controlled drug release systems and targeted drug delivery systems are two ways of describing these devices. Increased drug efficacy, site-specific administration, and reduced toxicity/side effects are only some of the therapeutic benefits of these Advance systems. Improved patient compliance, viable treatments for previously incurable diseases, the possibility of preventative applications, and greater ease of use are just a few of the benefits. Drug delivery systems lack a standard. In general, it is thought to depend on two factors: the route of administration (A) and (B) the dosage form. In this context, "drug delivery system" refers to any component of the Cartesian product (A x B) (**Figure 1**).

2. Drug delivery carriers

Vehicles for Drug Delivery: Micelle solutions, vesicle, liquid crystal dispersions, and nanoparticle dispersions comprising small particles between 10 and 400 nm in diameter are all examples of colloidal drug carrier systems that have shown significant promise as drug delivery methods. The objective of this kind of formulation development is to create substances with desirable characteristics, such as long shelf life, minimal toxicity, and optimum drug loading and release qualities. Incorporated drugs take part in the system's microstructure and may potentially affect it through molecular interactions, particularly if they have amphiphilic and/or mesogenic characteristics. The amphiphilic block copolymers' adaptability in terms of chemical composition, total molecular weight, and block length ratios, which permit regulation of the size and shape of the micelles, makes them desirable for use in drug administration applications. Block copolymers that have cross-linkable groups added to them can have their micelles stabilized and their temporal control enhanced. A very promising approach to a wider variety of locations of action with considerably higher selectivity is the substitution of block copolymer micelles with particular ligands.

3. Conventional methods of drug delivery

Pills, eye drops, ointments, and intravenous solutions are the standard methods of conventional drug administration. Numerous cutting-edge methods of administering drugs have emerged in recent years. Chemical drug modification, drug entrapment in macrovesicles for intravenous injection, and drug entrapment within pumps or polymeric materials for targeted delivery to specific anatomical sites are all examples of these methods (e.g., the eye or beneath the skin). These methods have already resulted in delivery systems that benefit human health, and further study has the potential to completely transform the way many medications are administered [11].

4. Evolution of drug delivery

The foundations for the study of drug release were laid between the years 1950 and 1980. The first generation of development occurred during this time, with controlled-release mechanisms being approved by regulatory bodies. For example, in 1952, the FDA approved Spansule (Smith, Kline, & French Laboratories), the first controlled-release drug delivery system. First-generation drug delivery methods relied on four primary drug-release mechanisms: controlled dissolution, controlled diffusion, controlled osmotic pressure, and controlled ion exchange [11]. There was some research into other processes, but from the 1950s to the 1980s, the majority of commercial products used a release mechanism based on dissolution, diffusion control, or a hybrid of the two. The majority of the time, these methods were used to administer drugs orally or topically. The second wave of drug delivery development began with injectables, with the approval of the first long-acting formulation in 1989. Originally developed to prolong the half-life of peptide and protein medications by a month, the poly (lactic-co-glycolic acid) (PLGA) microparticle formulation is an injectable depot formulation [12]. By adjusting the drug's ratio and molecular weight, the release time was lengthened to a full 6 months [4]. All other polymer-based long-acting injectable formulations have relied on PLGA for approval because of its proven safety. PEGylation, the technique by which poly (ethylene glycol) (PEG) is attached to protein molecules, is another important second-generation breakthrough [4]. By going through this procedure, protein molecules might remain in the body's bloodstream for a longer period of time. Subsequent research revealed a potential drawback, however, when antibodies were found to be formed within the body against the PEG molecules,

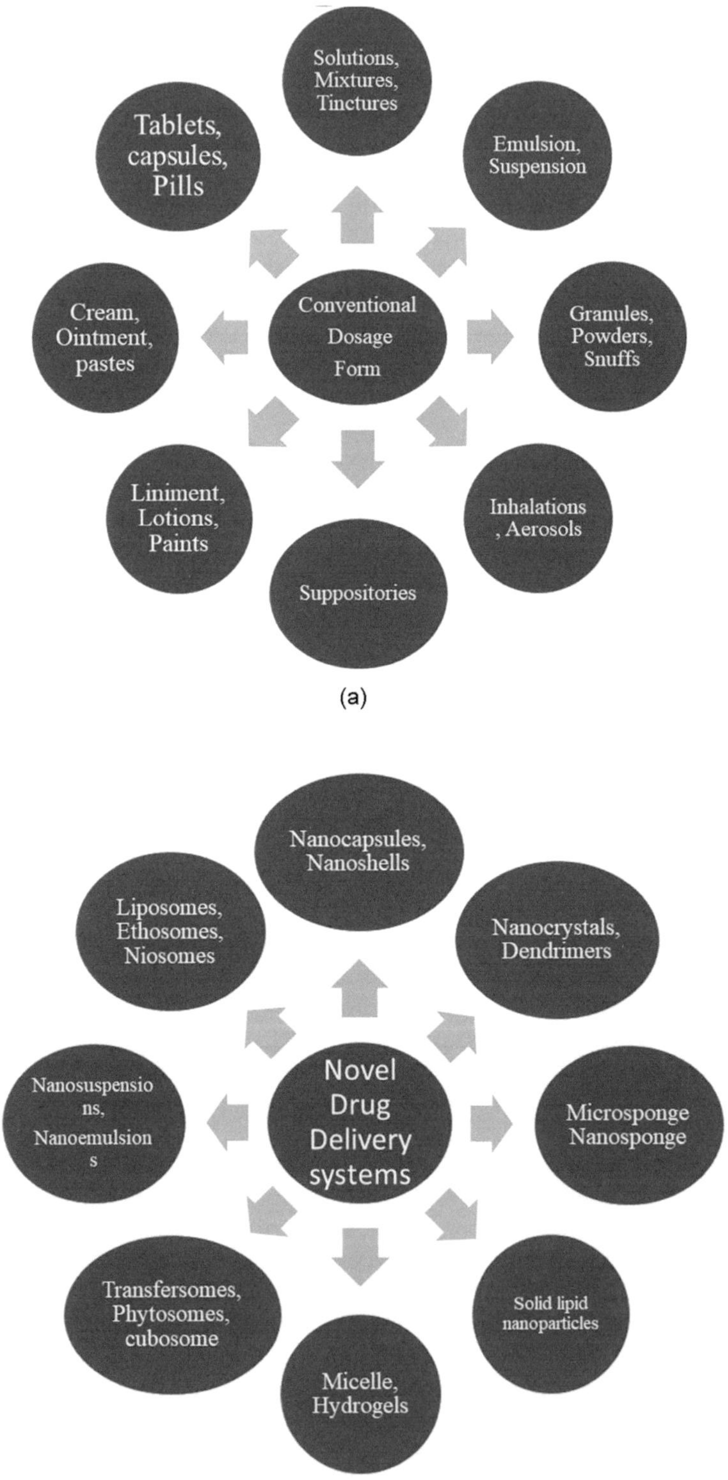

Figure 2.
(a) Conventional dosage forms (b) ADDS.

resulting in quicker blood clearance [5, 6]. PEGylation has to be better understood in order to be used more efficiently. PEGylation, and more especially lipid nanoparticles containing PEGylated lipid, has lately proven essential in the messenger RNA (mRNA) vaccines employed against COVID-19, which has sparked new interest in the field of lipid nanoparticles encapsulation and a Trojan Horse. Delivering mRNA vaccinations has been made practicable, something that was not conceivable when the medicinal application of mRNA vaccines was first proposed, some 30 years ago. This development has been brought to the forefront of world attention by the recent COVID-19 pandemic. In order to protect the vaccine molecules from the damaging effects of enzymes during transport, lipid nanoparticles must be encapsulated around the fragile mRNA. However, after the vaccine has been adequately shielded, it must be administered efficiently and exit the endosome before it can exert its therapeutic impact [4]. Due to decades of research, formulators were able to quickly construct an effective mRNA delivery system employing lipid nanoparticles during the COVID-19 pandemic. Scientists from Nanyang Technological University, Singapore, published a study into the use of conjugated peptide coacervates, a type of protein-based microdroplet, as a drug delivery vehicle for the intracellular administration of a wide variety of macromolecular therapeutics [13]. Therapeutics can enter cells via the protein-based microdroplets, which serve as a "Trojan Horse." Once the droplets have entered the cells, they breakdown, releasing the biomolecules that contain the drugs. The microdroplets are a useful vehicle for transporting many different types of medicines, including proteins, peptides, and messenger RNAs. The researchers also state that the microdroplets can be used to transport and administer a single or many macromolecular therapies (**Figure 2**) [13].

5. An evolving approach to drug delivery

Oral administration of an instantly active medicinal material has historically been the primary focus of medication delivery strategies. Due to the need for greater doses, the necessity for frequent administration, and the uncontrollable release of the therapeutic, the "traditional" modes of drug delivery have proven restricting for formulators as drug molecules have evolved and newer modalities have been researched. Because of this, bio/pharmaceutical firms have been putting a lot of effort into developing advanced drug delivery systems (ADDSs) to circumvent the drawbacks of current methods. The market trajectory for ADDS, which reflects the industry's attention, is predicted to develop at a compound yearly growth rate of 20.8% between 2021 and 2026, reaching an estimated value of $28.1 billion by the conclusion of the forecast period [14]. The advantages of controlled-release drug delivery, the existence of in vivo biological barriers that impact different properties of a drug substance, and the increased adoption of controlled-release drug delivery systems by certain patient populations due to non-adherence to treatment regimens are all factors that are expected to contribute to this growth [11, 15].

6. ADDS of herbal formulation

ADDS for herbal medications has received a lot of research and development attention in recent decades. There are two conditions that the unique carriers should ideally meet. The first requirement is that the drug is administered at a pace determined by the body's requirements during the course of treatment. Secondly, it needs to transport the herbal medicine's active ingredient to the affected area. None of these can be fulfilled by the standard or extended-release dose formulations currently available. Bioactive and plant extracts have been used in a wide range of innovative herbal formulations, including polymeric nanoparticles, nanocapsules, liposomes [16], phytosomes, nanoemulsions [17], microspheres [18], transferosomes, and ethosomes [19, 20]. In 2008, the advanced drug delivery systems industry was worth $134.3 billion worldwide, and in 2009, that number is expected to rise to $139 billion. The 2014 forecast of $196.4 billion represents a CAGR (over the next five years) of 7.2%. Targeted medication delivery is the largest market sector, with 2009 revenues of $50.9 billion and projected revenues of $80.2 billion in 2014, a CAGR of 9.5%. With projected revenues of $36.1 billion in 2009 and $45.8 billion in 2014, or a CAGR of 4.9%, sustained-release products hold the second greatest market share. In the case of drugs with a short half-life, sustained release can lead to less frequent dosing, improved compliance, and fewer fluctuations in plasma and blood levels, all of which contribute to a more reliable therapeutic effect [21, 22].

7. Conclusion

A new drug delivery system is an alternative to the conventional methods of administering drugs. In order to treat a patient, modern medicine first determines where in their body the disease is manifesting, and then delivers the medication directly to the area of the body where it will have the most effect. Poor bioavailability and plasma drug level variations characterize traditional drug delivery systems (tablets, capsules, syrups, ointments, etc.), rendering them incapable of achieving sustained release. Without a reliable method of administration, a treatment may as well not be attempted at all. Poor bioavailability and changes in plasma drug level characterize traditional drug delivery modalities (tablets, capsules, syrups, ointments, etc.). The entire therapy process may be ineffective without a reliable delivery method. Advanced drug delivery systems can be roughly categorized into three groups according to their intended use: rapid drug delivery, sustained drug delivery, and highly efficient drug delivery. Nanoparticles: The term "colloidal drug delivery system" refers to a broad category that includes nanoparticles. Microcapsules, nanocapsules, macromolecular complexes, polymeric beads, microspheres, liposomes, and niosomes are all types of encapsulation systems. Delivery of poorly soluble medicines and bioavailability difficulties for poorly soluble clinical candidates are major challenges in drug delivery systems. New methods have been developed for the transportation, surmounting of bioavailability barriers, and rational formulation design of poorly soluble medicines. There will be extensive use of NDDS in the treatment of chronic pain and other illnesses in the near future. Safety consciousness is evolving, and with that comes the necessity of narrowing in on a specific area to protect.

Author details

Sankha Bhattacharya[1], Paul Rodriques[2] and Bhupendra Prajapati[2]*

1 School of Pharmacy and Technology Management, SVKM'S NMIMS Deemed-to-be University, Shirpur, India

2 Shree S.K. Patel College of Pharmaceutical Education and Research Ganpat University, Mahesana, India

*Address all correspondence to: bhupen27@gmail.com; bhupendra.prajapati@guni.ac.in

References

[1] Tiwari G, Tiwari R, Sriwastawa B, Bhati L, Pandey S, Pandey P, et al. Drug delivery systems: An updated review. International Journal of Pharmaceutical Investigation. 2012;**2**(1e):2-11

[2] Patel R, Shah D, Prajapti BG, Patel M. Overview of industrial filtration technology and its applications. Indian Journal of Science and Technology. 2010;**3**(10):1121-1127

[3] Tamargo J, Le Heuzey JY, Mabo P. Narrow therapeutic index drugs: A clinical pharmacological consideration to flecainide. European Journal of Clinical Pharmacology. 2015;**71**(5):549-567

[4] Glassman PM, Muzykantov VR. Pharmacokinetic and pharmacodynamic properties of drug delivery systems. The Journal of Pharmacology and Experimental Therapeutics. 2019;**370**(3):570-580

[5] Vugmeyster Y, Xu X, Theil FP, Khawli LA, Leach MW. Pharmacokinetics and toxicology of therapeutic proteins: Advances and challenges. World Journal of Biological Chemistry. 2012;**3**(4):73-92

[6] Ulbrich K, Holá K, Šubr V, Bakandritsos A, Tuček J, Zbořil R. Targeted drug delivery with polymers and magnetic nanoparticles: Covalent and noncovalent approaches, release control, and clinical studies. Chemical Reviews. 2016;**116**(9):5338-5431

[7] Liechty WB, Kryscio DR, Slaughter BV, Peppas NA. Polymers for drug delivery systems. Annual Review of Chemical and Biomolecular Engineering. 2010;**1**:149-173

[8] Patel VM, Prajapati BG, Patel MM. Effect of hydrophilic polymers on buccoadhesive Eudragit patches of propranolol hydrochloride using factorial design. AAPS PharmSciTech. 2007;**8**(2):E119-EE26

[9] Patel RP, Patel MH, Prajapati BG, Baria AH. Formulation and evaluation of sustained release matrix tablet of tizanidine hydrochloride by direct compression technique. Journal of Science & Technology. 1 Jan 2011;**6**:69-81

[10] Patel SM, Patel RP, Prajapati BG. Solubility enhancement of benfotiamine, a lipid derivative of thiamine by solid dispersion technique. Journal of Pharmacy & Bioallied Sciences. 2012;**4**(Suppl. 1):S104

[11] Adepu S, Ramakrishna S. Controlled drug delivery systems: Current status and future directions. Molecules. 29 Sep 2021;**26**(19):5905. DOI: 10.3390/molecules26195905. PMID: 34641447; PMCID: PMC8512302

[12] Makadia HK, Siegel SJ. Poly lactic-co-glycolic acid (PLGA) as biodegradable controlled drug delivery carrier. Polymers. 2011;**3**(3): 1377-1397

[13] Sun Y, Lau SY, Lim ZW, Chang SC, Ghadessy F, Partridge A, et al. Phase-separating peptides for direct cytosolic delivery and redox-activated release of macromolecular therapeutics. Nature Chemistry. 2022;**14**(3):274-283

[14] Global Industry Analysts Inc. New analysis from global industry analysts reveals steady growth for novel drug delivery systems (NDDS), with the market to reach $28.1 Billion worldwide by 2026. Accessed December 3, 2022. Available from: https://www.prnewswire.com/news-releases/

new-analysis-from-global-industry-analysts-reveals-steady-growth-for-novel-drug-delivery-systems-ndds-with-the-market-to-reach-28-1-billion-worldwide-by-2026--301488680.html

[15] Yun YH, Lee BK, Park K. Controlled drug delivery: Historical perspective for the next generation. Journal of Controlled Release: Official Journal of the Controlled Release Society. 2015;**219**:2-7

[16] Bhattacharya S, Saindane D, Prajapati BG. Liposomal drug delivery and its potential impact on cancer research. Anti-Cancer Agents in Medicinal Chemistry (Formerly Current Medicinal Chemistry-Anti-Cancer Agents). 2022;**22**(15):2671-2683

[17] Macwan M, Prajapati B. Development, optimization and characterization of ocular nanoemulsion of an antifungal agent using design of experiments. Research Journal of Pharmacy and Technology. 30 May 2022;**15**(5):2273-2278

[18] Prajapati CV, Patel RP, Prajapati BG. Formulation, optimization and evaluation of sustained release microsphere of ketoprofen. Journal of Pharmacy & Bioallied Sciences. 2012;**4**(Suppl. 1):S101

[19] Bhokare SG, Dongaonkar CC, Lahane SV, Salunke PB, Sawale VS, Thombare MS. Herbal novel drug delivery: A review. World Journal of Pharmacy and Pharmaceutical Sciences. 2016;**5**(8):593-611

[20] Prajapati B. A review on PEGylated liposome in cancer therapy and in delivery of biomaterial. Pharmaceutical Reviews. 2007:5

[21] Prajapati BG, Solanki H. Recent techniques for oral time controlled pulsatile technology. The Internet Journal of Third World Medicine. 2009;**8**(1):1-23

[22] Patel DV, Prajapati BG. Preparation and evaluation of extended release pellets of chiral molecules of s-metoprolol succinate by different technology. Asian Journal of Pharmaceutics. 2017;**11**(3):210

Chapter 2

Advances in Natural Polymeric Nanoparticles for the Drug Delivery

Vikas Pandey, Tanweer Haider, Poornima Agrawal, Sakshi Soni and Vandana Soni

Abstract

Natural and biodegradable polymers have been the key area for utilizing their advantages which make them a possible option for development of various drug delivery systems. The complexity of diseases and the intrinsic drug toxicity and side effects has led to an interest for development and optimization of drug delivery systems. The advancements in nanotechnology have favored the development of novel formulations which can modulate the biopharmaceutical properties of bioactives and thus improves the pharmacological and therapeutic action. The shape, size, and charge nanoscale delivery system, such as nanoparticles (NPs) are required to be investigated and changed in order to promote and optimize the formulations. The various natural polymeric NPs (PNPs) have been found to be key tool to enhance bioavailability or specific delivery to certain site of action. In this chapter, the uses of various polymeric materials for the development of NPs as drug delivery systems for various ailments have been described. The entrapment of bioactive compounds in PNPs systems is a hopeful move toward improvement of efficacy of drug toward the treatments of various diseases.

Keywords: polymeric material, drug delivery, nanoparticles, targeting

1. Introduction

The research for natural polymeric material for the advancement in the drug delivery has been a prime focused for the researchers in the last two decades. The concept of natural polymeric material is one of the frontier research areas and is being focused for the enhancing the bioavailability along with the specific/targeted drug delivery and therapeutic index for the treatment of some life threatening diseases, like cancer [1]. Polymeric drug delivery system has been used to enable the delivery of drug molecule into the body for the therapeutic action. Various polymers biodegradable and non-biodegradable origin has been widely identified and used which are accompanying various advantageous features with them. For different novel drug delivery systems development, biodegradable and bio-reducible polymers are used which make a possible choice helping delivery of bioactives.

Nanotechnology is the branch which deals in the system, structures and devices in the range of nanometer. Nanotechnology has been a keen interest area in today's novel growing world associated with the significant development in controlled delivery of genes and drugs. NPs in the field of nanotechnology found to be very advantageous proving their efficiency for drug delivery, biodegradable nature, better bioavailability, versatility, less toxicity and high encapsulation efficiency. NPs carriers play a competent role for the controlled delivery of drug molecules for cancer therapy and site specific delivery of bioactive molecules as target site [2, 3].

The present chapter has complied the various natural polymeric material extensively used in the delivery of drugs and genes acting as the backbone for the development and delivery of bioactive agents in various cases.

2. Natural polymers for drug delivery

Natural polymers for the development of drug delivery and delivery of bioactive molecules have been extensively investigated producing better encapsulation of drugs, thus have attracted tremendous attention. These natural polymers do have the inherent advantages, such as biocompatibility, specific interactions with some biomolecules, controlled enzyme degradation, and easy surface modification furnish them with greater versatility in drug delivery. Different types of natural polymers and derivatives have been chemically and physically modified which are focusing the efficiently therapy through the use of various bioactive for smart stimuli-triggered or targeted delivery [4].

2.1 Animal-based biopolymers

2.1.1 Gelatin

Gelatin being a fibrous protein is identified as a natural, biocompatible, biodegradable, non-antigenic, low cost and multipurpose biopolymer and due to its unique mechanical and technological properties since timely memorial is commonly used in pharmaceutical (drug and vaccine delivery) cosmetic, food, and medical applications [5]. Gelatin is obtained from its parent molecule collagen in various thermo-reversible forms and the major commercial sources of gelatin are porcine or bovine skin, bones, aquatic and poultry sources [6]. But it has been observed that gelatin obtained from mammalian source is preferred over that produced from aquatic animal sources due to its strong gel strength, ideal gelling and melting temperatures, acceptable viscosity, and lack of fishy odor or allergens [7]. When gelatin is considered structurally it has triplets of the amino acids' alanine, proline, and glycine in repeating sequences that give gelatin its triple helical shape and both cationic and anionic groups chemically. It is this chemical composition of gelatin which is responsible for its stability and is exploited for chemical modification and covalent drug attachment in preparation of drug delivery systems [8]. These wide ranges of opportunities for chemical alterations and drug attachment of drug via covalent bond can be carried out either within the particle matrix or on the particle surface. In the former scenario, the gelatin macromolecules must undergo chemical alterations prior to the formation of NPs, whereas in the latter scenario, the particle surface is utilized [9].

Depending on its so easy to handle and play with availability of structure, it has been adapted for non viral gene delivery in various forms like alendronate gelatin,

PEGylated gelatin, cationic gelatin, thiolated gelatin, and EGFR gelatin NPs [10]. In context with these [11] designed MMP-2-triggered gelatin NPs loaded with doxorubicin (DOX) and 5-Aminolevulinic acid (5-ALA) providing combined chemotherapeutic and photodynamic therapy for breast cancer. The system employed the naturally occurring MMP-2 enzyme in tumor tissue, which via its high expression level was employed for gelatin degradation and targeted drug release was achieved [11]. Kirar et al. [12] found that a singlet oxygen was produced by biodegradable gelatin NPs damaging the microbial cell membrane, leading to cell death. The therapy regimen was adorned by Rose Bengal (RB) conjugated and entrapped in gelatin nanoparticle-based biodegradable nanophototheranostic. According to the study, gelatin NPs can be used in place of substances like potassium iodide, calcium chloride, ethylenediaminetetraacetic acid (EDTA), and polymyxin nonapeptide to allow drugs to penetrate cell membranes and exert antibacterial action [12].

2.1.2 Albumin

Albumin has been identified as most common protein in blood. Due to its function in the maintenance of intravascular colloid osmotic pressure, neutralization of toxins, high availability, non-immunogenic, strong binding capabilities for both hydrophobic and hydrophilic medicines, a lengthy half-life, the ability to target specific regions of inflammation, and almost little toxicity they have been readily accepted since the early twentieth century and welcomed for transport of therapeutic agents [13]. There are three forms of their existence and mainly utility is seen as bovine serum albumin, Human serum albumin, and Ovalbumin, [14]. The versatility of albumin-based NPs lies in their specificity been explored not only for deliverance of drugs but at the same time for navigating the possibilities of various drug delivery routes [15], multifunctional bioimaging [16], delivery of albumin functionalized aptamers [17–20] allowing its use as modified versions enhancing their interactions with enzymes like myeloperoxidases at inflamed site [21] achieving site specific drug delivery. In addition to these they are also utilized for conjugation with antibodies increasing their half life in circulation and was reported by [22] that engineered human albumin maintained FcRn-binding characteristics after conjugation and drop in glycemia was observed as a function of receptor targeting when given orally to human FcRn-expressing mice that had been given diabetes-inducing drugs, with a reduction up to 40% occurrence 1 h after delivery [22]. Albumin has also been explored for conjugation with nanobodies which are derived from different region of immunoglobulin's heavy chain single domain antibody [23]. Henaki et al. reported that a genetic fusion between the irrelevant nanobody R2 and the HER2-targeted nanobody 11A4 to increase binding with albumin-binding domain (ABD) leading to extended serum half-life noticeably, and uniform tumor formation [24].

2.1.3 Hyaluronic acid (HA) and its derivatives

HA is a natural polysaccharide discovered in 1934 from bovine eyes found in abundance as extracellular matrix's primary component, crucial to the human body's physiological processes. It is chemically composed of 1,3 and 1,4 glycosidic connections that frequently connect N-acetylglucosamine and glucuronic acid [25]. Since its discovery and further derivatization according to advances in drug delivery target potentials, improvisation of stability and shelf life is achieved. With these advancements, utility of HA and its derivatives in surgery, medication development, treatment of arthritis, targeting, formation of nanoparticulate/gel/microsphere/gene vectors based drug delivery systems has also enhanced over the past few years [26]. Bai et al. reported the construction of supramolecular self-assemblies of β-cyclodextrin and HA which were further drug–drug conjugates self-assembled into NPs for achieving active targeting. This multifunctional delivery system demonstrated co-drug delivery and release patterns that were responsive to pH and esterase, achieving improved synergistic therapeutic efficacy, and active targeting capability [27]. Hyaluronic acid mediated treatment possibility was checked by Lu et al., were by linking an o-phenylenediamine group, levofloxacin was conjugated with hyaluronic acid to create a CD44 mediated cellular targeting via NO-sensitive nano-micelles which provided with their ability to fight against bacteria leading to reduction in the inflammatory levels [28]. Duan et al., worked on coping up with thrombosis considered as one of the major complications of cancer by incorporating anticoagulant heparin (Hep) as an adjuvant to the therapy with carbon dots as drug delivery system loaded with doxorubicin hydrochloride. He found that this dual drug and adjuvant therapy enhanced the blood compatibility of the system and in vitro MTT and scratch tests showed that this drug delivery method could specifically suppress cancer cell growth and migration [29]. Hyaluronate mediated targeting of cancerous cell was also seen in breast cancer where Batool et al., create a papain grafted S-protected HA-lithocholic acid co-block (PAP-HA-ss-LCA) polymeric excipient that functions as an amphiphilic muco penetrating stabilizer for breast cancer epithelial cells. These cells are overexpressed with CD44 receptors. By creating a tamoxifen (TMX) loaded self-nanoemulsifying drug delivery system, the mucopermeating, stabilizing, and targeting capabilities of the PAP-HA-ss-LCA polymeric excipient were studied [30].

2.1.4 Silk fibroin

Polymer-based delivery systems that are effective must be biocompatible, biodegradable, low toxic, have the right mechanical properties, call for ambient production conditions, and offer sustained release. Due to its distinct structural characteristics of self-assembling capacity, high strength, processing flexibility, biodegradability, and biocompatibility, silk a natural polymeric biomaterial meet these needs [31]. A fibrous fundamental protein called Silk Fibroin (SF) and a stick-like coating made of sericin make up silk as it is well known. Commercially silk has been obtained from silk cocoons from silkworms of *Bombyx mori* mainly. Although Eight subspecies of Bombycoidea family, have been exploited but only the Bombycidae (mulberry) and Saturniidae (non-mulberry) are significant commercially [32]. According to descriptions of SF, it is a naturally occurring amphiphilic block co-polymer made up of hydro-phobic (highly conserved, arranged) and hydrophilic (less conserved, more complicated, less organized) blocks that combine to give SF its flexibility and strength. From a morphological perspective, SF consists of recurring chains made up of small side chain amino acids, such as glycine and alanine, and hydrophilic blocks having H-bonding and hydrophobic interactions, which are the basis of SF's tensile strength. Together with the less organized hydrophilic blocks, these effective hydrophobic blocks produce the flexibility [33, 34].

Cao et al., utilized FDA-approved SF, to utilize the advantages of the features as carrier polymer, demonstrating a single-step electrospraying procedure without an emulsion process uses the blends SF and polyvinyl alcohol (PVA) with drug. A distinct core-shell structure was obtained with doxorubicin encapsulated in the core.

By changing the PVA/SF ratio, the controlled drug release profiles were possible to achieve. The SF coating reduced the drug's first burst release, but a lot of drug molecules were still retained by the carrier polymers and portrayed a pH dependent drug release [35]. Chouhan et al., critically presented the use of SF in wound healing premises and showed the efficacy of silk based matrices for healing efficiency [36]. To overcome the problem of intravenous administration Gangrade et al., utilized two silk proteins and created a nano hybrid silk hydrogel-based delivery of anticancer medications locally, precisely, and instantly. The β-sheet structure helped to form the hydrogel network and payload efficiency was enhanced using the carbon nano tubes [37]. Air spun nanofibers for drug delivery [38], temperature-responsive poly (N-isopropylacrylamide) (PNIPAM) hydrogel and SF scaffold microcarriers for controlled and sustained drug release [39], silk based embolic material a potential next-generation multifunctional embolic agent including nivolumab labeled with albumin was delivered to treat vascular disorders, including malignancies, as well as achieve embolization [40]. Its utilization has been explored nevertheless in all possible directions for drug delivery.

2.2 Plant-based biopolymers

2.2.1 Cellulose

Cellulose is a high-molecular-weight natural homopolysaccharide, materialized as multifunctional drug delivery polymer because of their inbuilt porosity, which can aid in the liquid uptake. Water and cellulose can interact significantly, causing cellulose to swell easily in water. This swelling property is correlated with the cellulosic polymer network's capillarity. It is common knowledge that a medicine with a speedy swelling effect will also dissolve quickly and thus enhances the dissolution process [41]. Structurally cellulose connected to acetal molecule between the C-4 of hydroxyl group and C-1 of the carbon by covalent bond. One primary and two secondary hydroxyl groups can be found in anhydro glucose molecules. Because of the extremely strong inter- and intramolecular hydrogen bonds created by this hydroxyl group, cellulose is insoluble in aqueous or organic solvents. Cellobiose units are composed of two glucose moieties joined by a 1–4 bond having high molecular weight. D-hydroxyl glucose's is a good candidate for modification and the formation of various derivatives. Various derivatives of cellulose have been in use for various purposes depending on their physical properties like ethyl cellulose, methyl cellulose, carboy methyl cellulose, carboxy ethyl cellulose, hydroxy propyl methyl cellulose (HPMC), hydroxy ethyl cellulose, etc. [42]. Because of their properties they are used in ocular, rectal, vaginal, antitumor deliveries.

Recently, Long et al., recreated the efficacy of cellulose nanocrystals (CNCs) by utilizing the numerous hydroxyl active functional groups on the surface of CNCs allowing for easy chemical modification to improve targeting via manifesting weakly acidic tumor environment with a hydrazone bond along with anti-cancer drug. Owing to its properties Sheng et al., came up with $CaCO_3$ microspheres with methotrexate and aspirin co-entrapped in hydrogels, achieving significant pH dependent drug release on sites [43]. Pooresmaeil et al. [44], made use of Green chemistry to prepare layered double hydroxides LDHs known for their high ion exchangeability to deliver controlled and sustained drug release at acidic medium of stomach through loading of this LDH Zn/Al 5-Fluro uracil in CMC on site.

2.2.2 Starch

Starch, a readily available material, is most abundant and affordable biopolymer after cellulose and chitin that has been employed in a variety of biomedical applications, drug delivery systems, and tissue engineering platforms. Starch is a composition of two, amylose and amylopectin, which combine to generate these granules in chloroplast of plant cells. Amylose, a straight or slightly branched polysaccharide, is made up of glucose units connected by 1–4 glycosidic linkages while amylopectin is a branching biopolymer with extra -1-6 glycosidic linkages [45]. Shehabeldine et al. synthesized eco-friendly ciprofloxacin hydrochloride (CIP) loaded green-based nanocomposite to improve its activity and regulate the antibiotic's release and bioavailability. Microbiological glycoside hydrolases assist in the enzymatic hydrolysis of starch. Using an environmentally friendly process, hydrolyzed starch/chitosan loaded with CIP (HS/Ch-NC) was created. And optimal release of CIP was achieved [46]. A water soluble polysaccharide called as Pullulan is composed of maltotriose units and is produce by the fungus *Aureobasidium pullulans*, was reviewed by Grigoras for producing drug delivery systems enhancing therapeutic efficacy of hydrophobic drugs, increasing their water solubility [47]. Promoting the use of natural constituents for treatment purpose Nallasamy et al., designed a polyherbal nano-formulation incorporating Triphala churna in starch NPs exhibiting high loading efficiency, sustained release and its antibacterial, antibiofilm, and neuroprotective properties were equally retained [48].

2.2.3 Soy protein

After getting approved by UDFDA in 1999 as protective for coronary heart diseases its incorporation and utilization for various health treatments as adjuvants drastically increased. A globular protein extracted from soy beans, soy protein is relatively stable and has a long shelf life. Soy proteins when considered chemically have albumins and globulins as their primary components, which can be further segregated on the basis of sedimentation coefficients into 2S, 7S, 11S and even 15S fractions where 7S (SC), 11S (SG), or 15S fractions often correlate to the globulins, while the albumins in soy proteins are reported in the 2S form [49]. Mainly extracted from soy beans, they exist as soy flour, soy protein concentrate, and soy protein isolate available in quantities ranging from 50–90% after removal of carbohydrates, fats, oils, moisture and other components [50]. Its most commonly existing form is 11S (SG) consisting of 6 subunits. A disulfide bond connects the basic polypeptide (B) with the acidic polypeptide (A) that makes up each subunit. These subunits with functional groups like -NH_2, -OH, and -SH in soy protein make it easy to modify the protein chemically or physically or mix it with other biopolymers, which is equally reflected in the changes that the protein undergoes on heating, pH and other environmental exposures which are exploited for preparation of pH responsive gels, nano-formulations [51]. Being a good source of plant-based protein, it adds on formulations benefit in a way of being less immunogenic, more stable. They have a strong propensity to aggregate and gel, act as good emulsifiers, and are frequently employed as functional additives in food compositions. Its physical propensity has been identified with other plant-based ingredients like cellulose and pine needle extract for development of packaging material as well. Xu et al., by breaking the hydrogen bonds that existed between the N—H groups of soy proteins and water molecules added cellulose nanocrystals CNCs which reduced the moisture content, elongation at break of the film samples and increased the tensile strength as a result of the filling action of CNCs. Addition of pine extract not only added to antioxidant properties to the film but at the same time decreased its water permeability enhancing its water vapor barrier capacity [52]. Cheng et al. further advanced the drug release pattern and accumulation in cancer lines by grafting soya protein with D-α-Tocopheryl polyethylene glycol succinate which acted as an adjuvant to the Cisplatin delivery system by itself being a good stabilizer, wetting agent and solubilizer and provided acid responsive delivery [53]. Soy protein has been incorporated as 2D surfactant to enhance the electrical conduction of nanocomposites [54], as an excellent promoter of enzymatic hydrolysis extracted from inexpensive defatted soy powder (DSP) in liquid hot water pretreated lignocellulosic substrates making the process inexpensive and biocompatible [25, 55], as a 4D printing food material along with carrageenan, and vanilla as flavor enhancer [56].

2.2.4 Zein

First identified in nineteenth century, zein is a plant based prolamins extracted majorly from corn existing as α, β, γ, and δ zein. α zein ia considered the most common and abundant among existing varieties. It is a hydrophobic protein that dissolves better in aqueous acetone, aqueous ethanol, and various organic solvents other than in plain water. Being a hydrophobic protein, it is found to be suitable for drug delivery system designing due to its certain important features, like biocompatible, and biodegradable nature [57]. Its utility has been reported in multi-domains of pharmaceutical industry like food coating, packaging, tissue engineering as well. Various zein based delivery systems such as nanocarriers, microspheres, tablets, capsules electro-spun fibers, etc. for delivery of drugs in spatiotemporal manner has been used widely [58]. Manifesting its natural non immunogenic existence Ruberedo et al., reported preparation of PEG-coated zein NPs made by a simple and repeatable process without the use of reactive chemicals suitable for increasing the oral bioavailability of bioactives and other physiologically active substances with limited permeability [59]. The poor stability and re-dispersibility of zein NPs was mitigated by preparation of loading of anti-inflammatory drug imidazole into zeolitic imidazole framework-8 frame and further coating this with succinylated zein, these modifications were able to provide pH responsive oral delivery which was tested due to the stable under neutral conditions and rapidly degradation phenomenon in an acid environment due to protonation of zeolitic imidazole framework-8.

2.3 Biopolymers from marine organisms

2.3.1 Alginate

Alginates are polysaccharide polymers made up of sequence of two (1Ñ4)- linked α-L-guluronate (G) and β-D- (M) derived from brown seaweed (Phaeophyceae). They are biocompatible, show low toxicity and possess carboxyl groups which shows charge at pH values more than 3–4, making them soluble in alkaline and neutral environments. This pH dependent solubility portrayed by alginates and it's salts is promotive for some medications, for whom additional safeguards are required for preferential absorption in the lower gastrointestinal tract and thus are used to design various modified release dosage forms [60]. Santinon et al., reported delivery of Valsartan through sericin and alginate matrix, where addition of alginate during particle formation stage due to the gelation capacity on contacting with multivalent cations, such as Ca^{2+}, which helped in evaluating the efficacy of cross-linking agents like proanthocyanin, PVA, PEG, citric acid in formulations drug loading and drug release [61]. Properties of alginate to form pH sensitive gels was further extrapolated by Esfahlan et al., reported gelatin (Gel) and alginate (Alg) based a magnetic natural hydrogel, where after partly oxidizing alginate (OAlg), the Alg-Gel chemical hydrogel was created via a "Shift-Base" condensation process and then Fe_3O_4 magnetic NPs (MNPs) were entrapped into this gel via in situ chemical co-precipitation method. This resulted an efficient and "smart" drug delivery system for cancer chemotherapy as it out-performed free doxorubicin in terms of pH-dependent and delayed drug release profile, magnetic property for diagnosis by MRI approach, and isolation at targeted region [62]. They are utilized handsomely in pharmaceutical industry as thickening, gel-forming, and stabilizing properties whose action changes with concentration, environment/medium of dissolution involved [63].

2.3.2 Carrageenan

Carageenans discovered first in Ireland, are marine sourced linear polysachharides of red algae's that are sulphated [64]. Since 1973, the Food and Drug Administration (FDA) has deemed carageenans to be "Generally Recognized As Safe" (GRAS) (FDA SCOGS) (Select Committee on GRAS Substances). The European Food Safety Authority has certified carrageenan (E-407) and semi-refined carrageenan (E-407a) as food additives [65]. After receive of such approvals their inclusion in foods, pharmaceutical drug delivery systems increased. With time its efficiency has been seen in tissue engineering and regenerative medicines as well. Khan et al., designed porous polymeric nanocomposites and made use of sulphonic groups in carrageenan's structure which due to the self-assembly of their helical structures exhibit several biological properties along with acrylic-acid/graphene/hydroxyapatite. These nanocomposite scaffolds were able to enhance bone regeneration efficiently [66]. Vijaykumar et al., prepared zinc oxide NPs enveloped in kappa-carrageenan for anti-inflammatory effects on Methicillin resistant *Staphylococcus aureus* (MRSA) culture, where this MRSA causes human skin and nosocomial infections. The formulation acted as super bug for MRSA growth at a minimal concentration, reducing bacterial cell surface hydrophobicity with no evidence of hemolytic or morphological changes in human RBC [67]. It has been reported that sulphated algae polysaccharides showed anti-viral activity for which carrageenan and fucoidan where considered the norms for viral crisis of which kappa carrageenan with higher sulphated content proved to be really effective [68].

2.3.3 Chitosan

Chitosan is a linear naturally occurring amino polysaccharide, Rouget made the initial discovery and discussion of it in 1859 revealing its generation from chitin. After celluloe, chitosan is considered to be the second most prevalent amino polysaccharide after cellulose. Significant research has been conducted on pharmaceutical and bio-medical and applications, such as drug delivery, tissue engineering, wound-healing dressing, etc. because of its nontoxic, biocompatible, antibacterial, and biodegradable qualities. It is structurally made up of repeated glycosidic units made of *N*-acetyl-D-glucosamine and D-glucosamine units, each of which has two hydroxyl groups and one amino group. The amino group which carve out for the cationic versatility of chitosan to provide rate and time specific drug release, bio-adhesion, in situ gelation, antibacterial, permeation enhancement, etc. [69]. Chitosan can be classified according to its inherent features, such as purity, molar mass, viscosity, acetylation level, quality, and physical shape. Chitosan's performance, synthesis, characterization, and applications are all influenced by its degree of acetylation characteristics as well as its molar mass [70]. Baghaei et al., prepared a polyelectrolyte complex of trimethyl chitosan, hyaluronate/dextran/alginate NPs using D optimal design and checked their efficacy for gene delivery and for further translational work in industries. He found that chitosan and hyaluronate showed desired size, entrapment efficiency and in-vitro killing [71]. Ziminska et al., in line of promoting the patient compliance, a thermo responsive gel was designed for minimal invasive delivery utilizing free radical polymerization to create a stable, hydrogel network at body temperature, with low molecular weight chitosan of 75–85% deacetylation and *N*-isopropylacrylamide with unique physical characteristics were used. The fact that NCTC-929 cells could be transfected by the released RALA/pEGFP-N1 indicates that the hydrogel had no effect on the stability of the supplied nucleic acid [72].

2.3.4 Fucoidan

Enormous marine supply of ingredients showing biocompatibility, non-immunogenicity, and bioavailability has increased their demand in numerous fields, including biology, food science, pharmacology and cosmetics, empowering the value of this resource. Three major categories of marine biomaterials are as follows: lipids, polysaccharides, and proteins [73]. Out of these three biomaterials, marine polysaccharides are most stable, with fundamental or covalent structure which shows the arrangement of monomeric units throughout the chain which are used to categorize them. By restricting the orientations of the monomers, these repeating units are joined by covalent chemical bonds. This property limits the forms that a polysaccharide chain may take on, known as "secondary structures". Depending on these fundamental sequences marine polysaccharides possess inherent qualities that are extremely important in the field of medication delivery. Biomaterials utilizing enzymatic and chemical processes, developing stimuli-responsive delivery vehicles, modified as gels, and produce interpenetrated polymeric networks [74]. These may further get conjugated, and complexes with bioactive molecules or proteins [75]. Fucoidan is one such marine sulfated polysaccharide obtained from brown algae and invertebrates from marine origin. A top-notch candidate for pharmaceutical uses is fucoidan. Because of its many biological features, including antiviral, anticoagulant, antiangiogenic, anticancer, antioxidant, antiproliferative, anti-inflammatory, and immunomodulating activities, fucoidan has recently received attention [76]. For instance, fucoidan's anticancer action is mostly associated with its lower molecular weight [77]. Shanmugapriya et al., designed fucoidan-based nanomaterials for the precise medicine administration to the cancer cells in the gastrointestinal tract loaded with nanohydroxyapatite/collagen. The formulation showed effective results with potent administration of drug at target site [78].

3. Natural PNPs for cancer nanomedicine

As cancer is becoming the main cause of mortality in wealthy nations. In fact, according to specialists, there will be a 70% increase in the occurrence of this disease during the next 20 years [79, 80]. Surgery, chemotherapy, and radiation make up the standard treatment regimen for treating cancer. The most general form of cancer treatment is chemotherapy, but it has a high level of toxicity since it affects both healthy and malignant cells [81]. An option that is more focused is known as "nanomedicine," which is the use of materials at the nanometric scale in medicine. Its primary goal in oncology is to deliver the medication solely to cancer cells in order to increase its efficacy and lessen its toxicity. Additionally, early cancer detection technologies and combination medicines that improve treatment effectiveness and prognosis are both possible applications of nanomedicine [80]. Many PNPs have been employed up to this point to transport anticancer medications like paclitaxel, doxorubicin, or camptothecin in various cancers. By experimenting with new drug delivery methods, mixing active ingredients to enhance their effects, or combining with other therapies like gene therapy, the usage of PNPs can lead to advancements in cancer treatment. As an alternative to intravenous delivery, Ahmad et al. [82] suggested improving the oral bioavailability of doxorubicin by surface-modified biodegradable PNPs. They investigated the pharmacokinetics of doxorubicin and drug-loaded PEGylated PLGA NPs in Wistar rats. Results indicated that when compared to oral medications, NPs had superior activity and higher bioavailability. Soma et al. [83] investigated the synergistic impact of doxorubicin and cyclosporin A nanoparticulate formulations in comparison to NPs alone is successful in slowing the growth rate of P388/ADR cells, according to the results. The FDA has authorized albumin-bound (nab)-paclitaxel NPs (Abraxane®) for the treatment of cancer in 2012. Since then, a wide range of cancers, including pancreatic cancer, metastatic breast cancer, and lung carcinoma have been treated with it. These NPs were created to help with paclitaxel's pharmacokinetics and pharmacodynamics as well as to prevent the toxicities of the polyoxyethylated castor oil solvent (Cremophor), which was previously employed since paclitaxel had a difficult time dissolving in water. Additionally, these NPs plus gentamicin together had a somewhat higher survival probability for advanced and metastatic pancreatic cancer. A new paclitaxel liposome-albumin composite that was recently developed at the nanoscale had a remarkable encapsulation effectiveness of 99.8% [84].

Brain Targeted PNPs were also investigated by researchers and to be found affective drug delivery. Crpanl et al. [85] investigated camptothecin-loaded cyclodextrin NPs for brain cancer. The effectiveness of these NPs demonstrated an increase in the survival time and was studies in a rat glioma model for brain cancers. Pandey et al., reported the improved delivery of anticancerous agent doxorubicin via surface modified silk fibroin NPs through Tween-80 coating. The hydrophobic nature of these NPs assists make then susceptible for macrophageal and reticulo-endothelial system (RES) uptake which was overcome by surface coating of NPs with Tween-80 which is a hydrophilic stabilizers, thus making them long circulating and helping to cross blood brain barrier (BBB) by low density lipoprotein (LDL) [34].

Breast cancer, most common kind of cancer in women, is accounting for a staggering 30% of all instances that have been officially diagnosed. In order to better understand the effects of pH-sensitive PEG-PLGA-PGlu (polyglutamic acid) NPs implanted with doxorubicin and curcumin on breast tumor cells and drug-resistant cancer stem cells, Yuan et al. used mouse models [86]. Hu et al. looked at the usage of photodynamic therapy and nanoparticulate systems together in the treatment of breast cancer. They created oxygen-producing theranostic poly(caprolactone-co-lactide)-b-PEG-b-poly(caprolactone-co-lactide) NPs of doxorubicin, chlorin e6, and colloidal MnO_2 to create oxygen in tumor environment, relieve tumor hypoxia, and enhance photodynamic therapy. The NPs also improves the action of doxorubicin [87]. Breast cancer has also been studied in relation to MDR.

As the third cause of death brought on by oncologic diseases, liver cancer is the most common malignancies with high mortality rate. The majorities of anti-cancer medications have considerable liver toxicity and can result in serious adverse effects. With the aim of to increase the efficiency of anticancer medications and to lessen the emergence of adverse effects, PNPs are used as potential carriers. Zhu et al. reported a novel galactosamine-conjugated polydopamine-modified copolymer (Gal-pD-TPGS-PLA) NPs to create a nanosystem [88]. Gal-pD-TPGS-PLA NPs was used to target HepG2 cells by ASGP receptor-mediated recognition, and dramatically decrease cell growth, according to an in vitro cellular uptake and cytotoxicity study. Furthermore, docetaxel-loaded Gal-pD-TPGS-PLA NPs decreased tumor growth more as compared to docetaxel-loaded TPGS-PLA NPs, pD-TPGS-PLA NPs, or saline, in vivo. An overview of the nanoparticulate systems used as drug delivery system for cancer therapy are summarized in **Table 1**.

Biactive	Polymer	Type of cancer	Experimental model	References
Camptothecin	PCL–PEG	Glioma	4 T1 cells in BALB/c mice	[85]
Docetaxel	Gal–pD–TPGS–PLA	Liver Cancer	MCF-7 cells in BALB/c mice	[88]
Docetaxel and salinomycin	TPGS–PLGA	Breast Cancer	MCF-7/DOX cell line	[89]
Doxorubicin	PEGylated PLGA	Various	Bioavailability assay in Wistar rat	[82]
Doxorubicin and Chlorin e6 MnO2	PCLLA–PEG–PCLLA	Breast Cancer	MCF-7/ADR cells xenograft in female BALB/c nude mice	[87]
Doxorubicin and metformin	TPGS–PLGA	Breast Cancer	MCF-7 cells in nude mice	[90]
Doxorubicin–curcumin	mPEG–PLGA–PGlu	Breast Cancer	LM2 cells in BALB/c homozygous nude mice	[86]
Doxorubicin–cyclosporin A.	PACA	Various	P388/ADR cells line	[83]
Paclitaxel	Lip–BSA	Various	4T1 cells in BALB/c mice	[84]
Paclitaxel	PLGA–PEG	Glioma	Gliosarcoma 9L cells in Fischer F344 rats	[89]
Paclitaxel	PLA–PEG–maleimide	Breast Cancer (TNB)	MDA-MB-231 cells BALB/c homozygous nude mice	[86]
Paclitaxel	PCL–PEGPEG–PCL	Lung Cancer	MCF-7/ADR cells in BALB/c nude mice	[87]
Paclitaxel	PEI–PLA	Lung Cancer	A549 cells in BALB/c mice	[91]

Table 1.
Polymeric NPs bearing anticancer drug for cancer treatment.

4. Methods of preparations for PNPs

Methods of preparations for PNPs are classified as general methods and modern methods which are discussed in details as follow.

4.1 General methods

Recently, various biodegradable polymers and their co-polymers have been used to create NPs, being the most frequently used to create PNPs and encapsulate bioactive. Micelles, platelets, dendrimers, fibers, spheroids colloids, core-shells, and polymer matrixes with embedded NPs are just a few examples of multi-functionalized polymeric nanocarrier systems (**Figure 1**).

Depending on the specific application, PNPs must have their characteristics tuned. The method of preparation is crucial in achieving the desired qualities. Consequently, it is very beneficial to have preparation methods on hand in order to create PNPs with the appropriate characteristics for a certain application. Various methods are employed, including polymerization, premade polymers, ionic gelation, etc. These can be completed using the many techniques listed below.

- Solvent evaporation
- Nanoprecipitation
- Emulsification/solvent diffusion
- Salting out
- Dialysis
- Supercritical fluid technology (SCF).

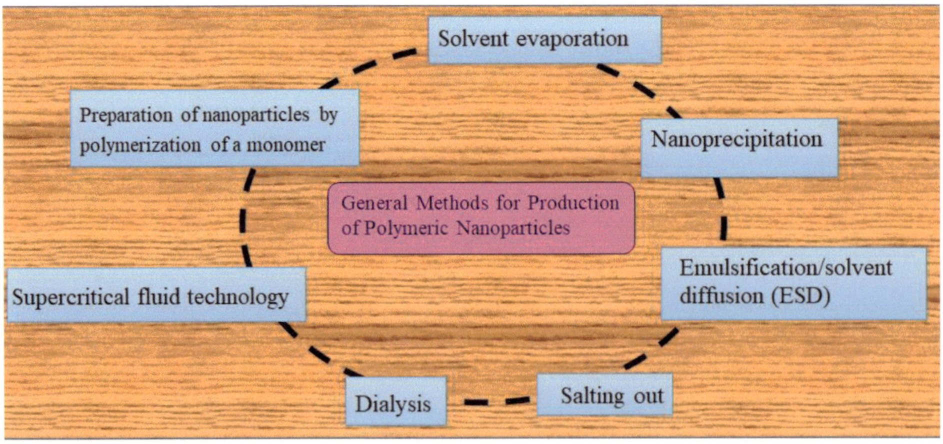

Figure 1.
General methods of preparation of PNPs.

Methods for preparation of NPs from polymerization of monomers

- Emulsion
- Mini emulsion
- Micro emulsion
- Interfacial polymerization
- Controlled/Living radical polymerization (C/LRP)
- Ionic gelation or coacervation of hydrophilic polymers

4.1.1 Solvent evaporation

The first technique created to make PNPs was solvent evaporation. This method involves development of polymer solutions in volatile solvents and creating emulsions. Ethyl acetate, which has a superior toxicity profile, has replaced dichloromethane and chloroform premade polymer [92], which were once frequently utilized. As the solvent evaporates and allowed to pass into the continuous phase of the emulsion, the emulsion is transformed into a suspension of NPs. The manufacture of single-emulsions, such as oil-in-water (o/w) or double-emulsions, such as w/o/w, are the two major techniques utilized in the conventional procedures for creating emulsions. These techniques involve ultrasonication or high-speed homogenization, followed by the solvent evaporation either by continuous magnetic stirring at ambient temperature or under decreased pressure. NPs can be recovered by ultracentrifugation and rinsed with distilled water to get rid of additives (**Figure 2**). The product is lyophilized at the end [92, 93].

4.1.2 Nanoprecipitation

Solvent displacement technique is another name for nanoprecipitation. A polymer from organic solution gets precipitated, and the organic solvent diffuses across the

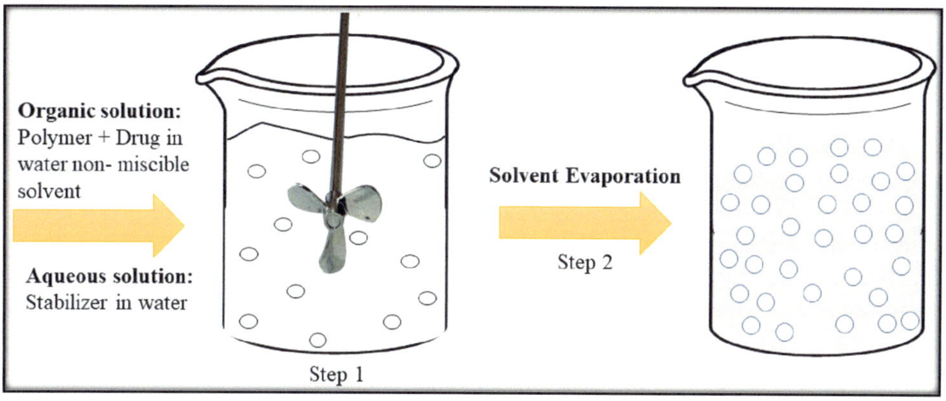

Figure 2.
Solvent-evaporation technique for NPs formation.

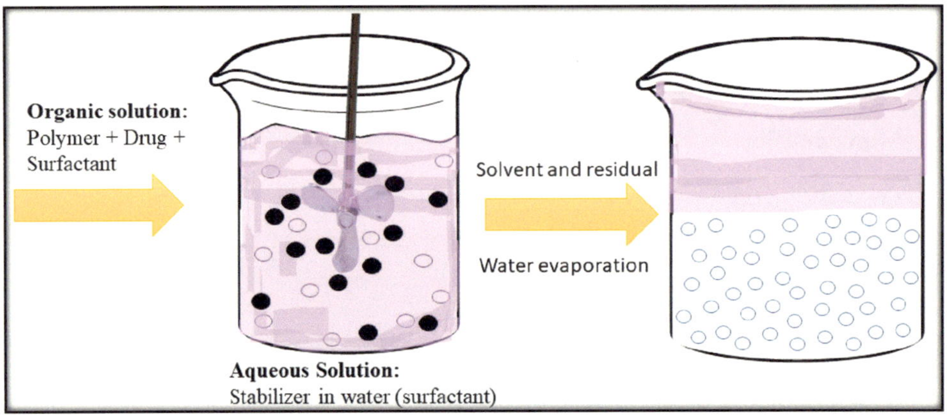

Figure 3.
Nanoprecipitation technique (surfactant is optional) for NPs formation.

aqueous medium whether a surfactant is present or not [94, 95]. The nanospheres precipitation occurs for the polymer, typically PLA, which get dissolved in a water-miscible solvent (medium polarity). This phase is added to an aqueous solution with agitation and contains a stabilizer as a surfactant. Instantaneous production of a colloidal suspension results from polymer deposition on the water-organic solvent interface brought on by the solvent's rapid diffusion [96]. Phase separation is carried out using a fully miscible solvent that is also a non-solvent of the polymer to help the production of colloidal polymer particles during the first step of the operation [97]. Although acetone and dichloromethane (ICH, class 2) are employed to dissolve and enhance drug entrapment, the dichloromethane increases mean particle size [98], and it is therefore hazardous. Due to the solvent's miscibility with the aqueous phase, this approach can only be used to encapsulate lipophilic pharmaceuticals and is ineffective for water-soluble medications. Numerous polymeric polymers, including PLGA, PLA, PCL, and poly (methyl vinyl ether-comaleic anhydride) (PVM/MA), have been subjected to this technique [99, 100]. Entrapment efficiencies of up to 98% showed that this method was well suited for the inclusion of cyclosporin A [101]. The antifungal medications Bifonazole and Clotrimazole were loaded into nanoparticulate systems using the solvent displacement approach (**Figure 3**) [102].

4.1.3 Emulsification/solvent diffusion (ESD)

A modified form of the solvent evaporation technique is used here [103]. To attain the initial thermodynamic equilibrium of liquids phase, the polymer gets dissolved in a slightly water soluble solvent, like propylene carbonate. It is necessary to encourage the diffusion of the dispersed phase's solvent by dilution with an excess of water which results in the formation of precipitate of the polymer and the subsequent NPs formation. Then, depending on the ratio of oil to polymer, the polymer-water solvent phase is emulsified in an aqueous solution with stabilizer, resulting solvent diffusion to exterior phase leading to the formation of nanocapsules or nanospheres (**Figure 4**). Depending on its boiling point, the solvent is finally removed via evaporation or filtering. **Figure 4** shows the process in action. The mesotetra(hydroxyphenyl)porphyrin- and doxorubicin-loaded PLGA (p-THPP) NPs, the plasmid DNA- and coumarin-loaded PLA NPs, the indocyanine- and the cyclosporine (Cy-A)-loaded gelatin- and sodium glycolate-loaded NPs were NPs developed by the ESD technique (**Figure 4**) [104].

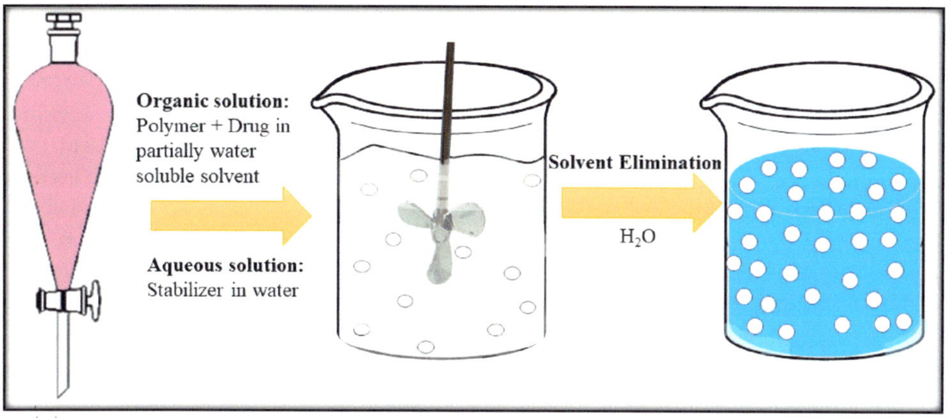

Figure 4.
Emulsification/ solvent diffusion technique for NPs formation.

4.1.4 Salting out

The principle behind salting out is the use of the salting out phenomenon to separate a water miscible solvent from aqueous solution. A variant of the emulsification/solvent diffusion process is the salting out process. The salting-out agent such as electrolytes (calcium chloride, magnesium chloride, etc) or non-electrolytes (sucrose) and a colloidal stabilizer (PVP or hydroxyethyl cellulose) are added to the initially dissolved polymer and drug is dissolved in a solvent, like acetone. This o/w emulsion is thinned out with enough aqueous solution to speed up acetone's diffusion into the liquid phase, which causes the production of nanospheres [93]. Salting out agent selection is crucial since it can have a significant impact on how effectively the medicine is encapsulated (**Figure 5**). To remove both the solvent and salting out agent, cross-flow filtration is used. This method is very effective and simple to scale up. Salting out has the principal benefit of reducing stress on protein encapsulants [105]. When heat-sensitive materials need to be treated, salting out may be helpful because it does not need a rise in temperature [106].

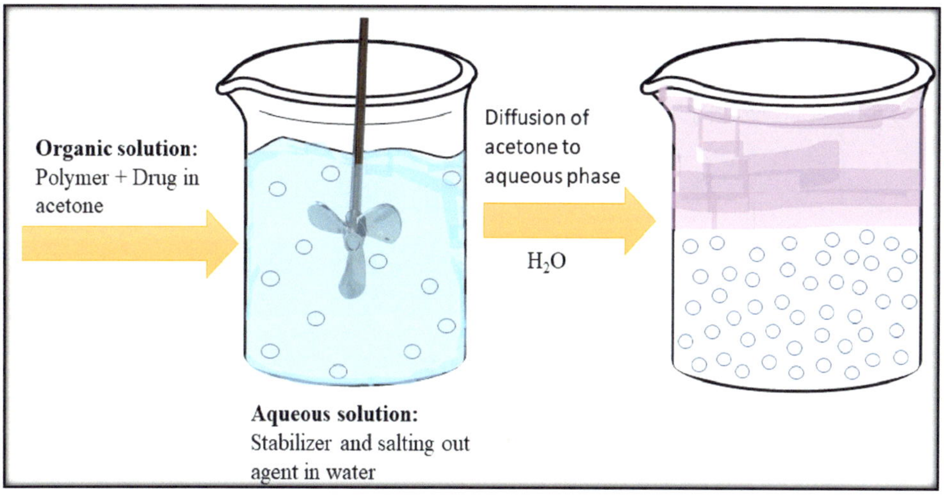

Figure 5.
Salting out technique for NPs formation.

4.1.5 Dialysis

Small, narrow-distributed NPs can be produced using a quick and efficient procedure called dialysis [107–109]. A dialysis tube is filled with a polymer dissolved in an organic solvent and has had the appropriate molecular weight cut off. Another non-solvent miscible with the solvent is used for dialysis. The polymer gradually gets aggregates as a result of decrease in solubility leading to development of homogenous NPs suspensions. The shape and size of NPs are influenced by type of solvent evolve to make the polymer solution. For the manufacture of different natural and synthetic PNPs, Chronopoulou et al. [110] developed a unique osmosis-based technique (**Figure 6**). This method is based on physical barrier (dialysis membrane or semi-permeable membranes) which enable the passive transit of solvents resulting decelerate the mixing process of non-solvent with polymer. The polymer solution presents in the dialysis membrane.

4.1.6 Supercritical fluid technology

The use of supercritical fluids technology is more environmentally friendly having the power to produce the highly pure PNPs without any traces of organic solvent [111]. With the majority of the limitations of conventional approaches avoided, supercritical fluid technology and dense gas technology are predicted to offer an intriguing and efficient method of particles creation.

For the synthesis of NPs with supercritical fluids, two concepts have been developed:

1. Rapid expansion of supercritical solution (RESS).

2. Rapid expansion of supercritical solution into liquid solvent (RESOLV).

4.1.6.1 Rapid expansion of supercritical solution

RESS involves dissolving the solute in a supercritical fluid to create a solution, which is then rapidly expanded over an aperture or a capillary nozzle into the surrounding air. The creation of well-dispersed particles is caused by homogeneous nucleation. For homogeneous nucleation, the high degree of super saturation and

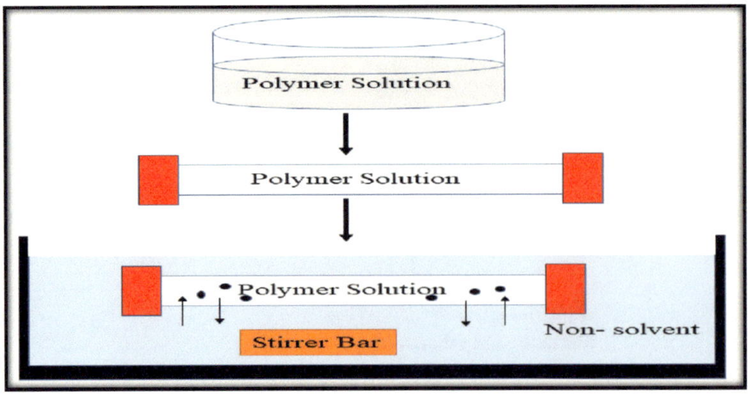

Figure 6.
Osmosis-based method for polymer NPs formation.

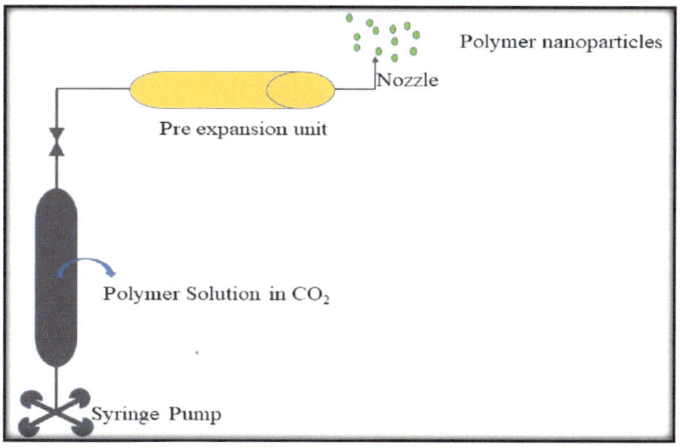

Figure 7.
RESS method for polymer NPs formation.

quick pressure reduction in the expansion are the requirements. Both nanometer and micrometer sized particles are able to get produced through expansion jet. Three main components of the RESS experimental equipment are (a) high pressure stainless steel mixing cell, (b) a syringe pump, and (c) a preexpansion unit. At room temperature, a polymer solution in CO_2 is created. Syringe pumps are used to pump the solution to the pre-expansion unit where it is isobarically heated to the pre-expansion temperature before it leaves the nozzle. Now, at atmospheric pressure, the supercritical solution is left to expand through the nozzle (**Figure 7**). For RESS, the particle size and shape are significantly influenced by the polymer's concentration and saturation level [112, 113].

4.1.6.2 Rapid expansion of supercritical solution into liquid solvent

Expansion of the supercritical solution into solvent rather than ambient air is a straightforward but important adjustment to the RESS process [106]. Poly (heptadecafluorodecyl acrylate) NPs having size less than 50 nm were created. Although, there is no organic solvents involvement in the RESS process for the formation of PNPs, still the fundamental disadvantage of RESS is that the primary products created using this technique are microscaled rather than nanoscaled. A new supercritical fluid technique called RESOLV has been created to get over this limitation. The liquid solvent in RESOLV inhibits particle development in the expansion jet, allowing the formation of mostly nanosized particles (**Figure 8**) [114].

4.1.7 NPs formation by polymerization of a monomer

Designing appropriate polymer NPs can be done during the polymerization of monomers in order to get the needed characteristics for a specific application. The procedures for creating PNPs by polymerizing monomers are explained below.

4.1.7.1 Emulsion polymerization

The quickest and most scalable process for producing NPs is emulsion polymerization. Depending on whether an organic or an aqueous continuous phase is used, the approach is grouped into two groups. In order to use the continuous organic phase

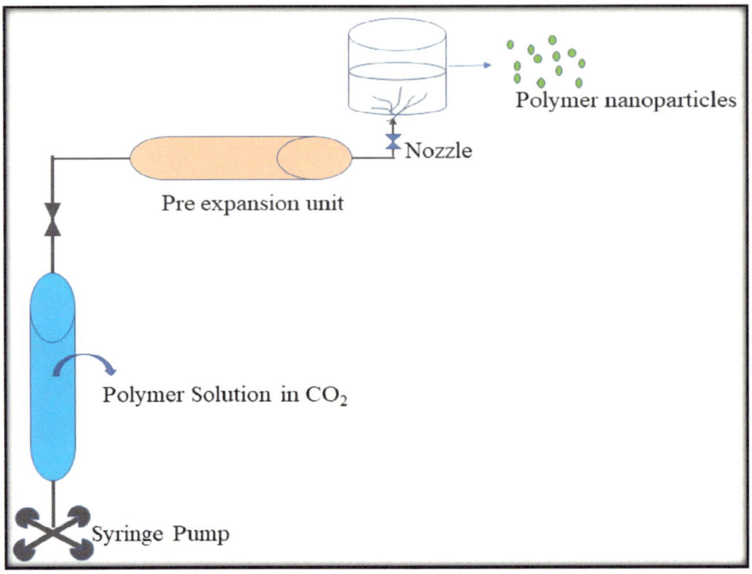

Figure 8.
RESOLV process.

approach, a monomer must be dispersed into an emulsion, an inverse microemulsion, or a substance in which it is not soluble (nonsolvent). Using this technique, polyacrylamide nanospheres were created [115]. Later, via dispersion of surfactants into solvents including cyclohexane, n-pentane, and toluene as the organic phase, poly(ethylcyanoacrylate) (PECA), poly(methylmethacrylate) (PMMA), and poly(butylcyanoacrylate) (PBCA) NPs were generated. Surfactants or emulsifiers are not required in the dissolving continuous aqueous phase. When a monomer molecule get dispersed in continuous phase, it strikes an initiator molecule (may be ion or a free radical) initiation starts. As an alternative, powerful ultraviolet or visible light, high-energy radiation can convert the monomer molecule to act as an initiating radical. According to an anionic polymerization process, chain development begins when starting monomer ions or radicals strike additional monomer molecules. Before or after the polymerization process has finished, phase separation and the production of solid particles may occur [116].

4.1.7.2 Mini-emulsion polymerization

Water, a monomer combination, a costabilizer, a surfactant, and an initiator make up a typical formulation for miniemulsion polymerization. Differences between mini-emulsion polymerization and emulsion polymerization is the use of a high-shear device and a low molecular mass molecule which act as co-stabilizer (ultrasound, etc.).

4.1.7.3 Micro-emulsion polymerization

A novel and successful method for producing PNPs has gained a lot of attention: micro-emulsion polymerization. The emulsion and micro-emulsion polymerization techniques are involved in the formation of colloidal polymeric particles via using completely different kinetic. Micro-emulsion polymerization technique results in much lower particle sizes. A thermodynamically stable micro-emulsion with swollen micelles is introduced to the aqueous phase of micro-emulsion polymerization together with water-soluble initiator. The polymerization starts from this spontaneously point which help in production of thermodynamically stable state which depends on large amounts of surfactant complexes having almost zero interfacial tension at the o/w contact. Additionally, due to the application of surfactant in high amount, the particles are totally covered by surfactant. The delicate micro-emulsions are later destabilized by the elastic and osmotic impact of the chains, which generally result in a rise in particle size, the generation of empty micelles, and subsequent nucleation. In the finished product, the bulk of empty micelles coexist with very tiny latexes, with size of about 5–50 nm. Some of the key variables influencing the kinetics and characteristics of PNP in microemulsion polymerization techniques are the type and concentrations of the initiators, surfactant, monomer, and reaction temperature [117].

4.1.7.4 Interfacial polymerization

It is one of the tried-and-true techniques for creating polymer NPs. The reaction for the process occurs at the interface of the two liquids. It utilizes the polymerization as step by step process of two reactive monomers that are distributed in two phases, respectively. By using interfacial cross-linking processes (polyaddition, polycondensation, radical polymerization) nanometer-sized hollow polymeric particles were formed [118]. By polymerizing monomers at the o/w interface of o/w micro-emulsion, oil-containing nanocapsules were created. It was thought that the interfacial polymerization of the monomer took place at the surface of the oil droplets which was formed during emulsification and organic solvent (miscible with water) functioned as a monomer carrier. Aprotic solvents like acetone and acetonitrile should be used to encourage the development of nanocapsules [119].

4.1.8 Controlled/living radical polymerization

Future commercial success of controlled/living radical polymerization depends on its application in the industrially significant aqueous dispersion systems, which produces PNPs having control over particle size and size distribution. Atom transfer radical polymerization (ATRP), reversible addition and fragmentation transfer chain polymerization (RAFT), and Nitroxide-mediated polymerization (NMP) are some of the successful in-depth approaches for controlled/living radical polymerization that are now accessible [120]. Hydrophilic polymers may gel or accelerate ionically. Some biodegradable hydrophilic polymers like gelatin, sodium alginate, and chitosan are generally used for the development of PNPs. By using ionic gelation, a technique for producing hydrophilic chitosan NPs was developed. Ionic gelation was used to create chitosan NPs that were loaded with dexamethasone sodium phosphate [121]. Chitosan is a di-block co-polymer of ethylene oxide or propylene oxide (PEO-PPO), and poly anion sodium tripolyphosphate are the two aqueous phases that are mixed together in the procedure. Through the interaction with the negatively charged tripolyphosphate, positively charged amino groups of chitosan forms coacervates of size range in nanometer. In contrast to ionic gelation, which occurs when a substance changes from a liquid to a gel as a consequence of ionic interaction conditions at ambient temperature, coacervates are created via electrostatic contact between two aqueous phases. Ionic gelation method for formation of PNPs is shown in **Figure 9**.

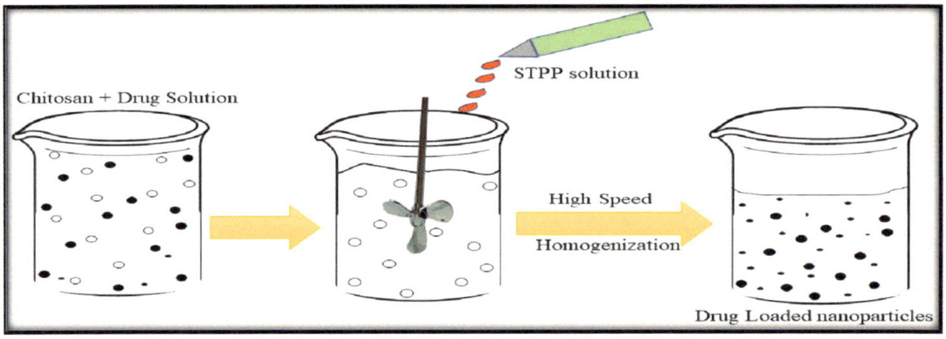

Figure 9.
Ionic gelation method for formation of PNPs.

4.2 Modern methods

The recognition of the multi-functional, environment-responsive, targeted, and controlled drug delivery system has recently made PNPs as one of the most promising and practical technological platforms. In a rapidly developing new technical field called "polymer in smart medication delivery", many therapeutic uses of nanotechnology are anticipated to address patient concerns in the medical field.

The use of several contemporary techniques, including microelectromechanical systems [122], microfluidic systems [123], electrodropping system [77], advanced high pressure homogenization, microneedle based system, interfacial emulsion polymerization, etc. are helpful to synthesize a variety of novel biocompatible polymers with well-defined nanometers to a few micrometers structures. The few contemporary methods for creating PNPs are shown in **Figure 10**. Based on the particular application, the physiochemical properties of PNPs must be tuned. To

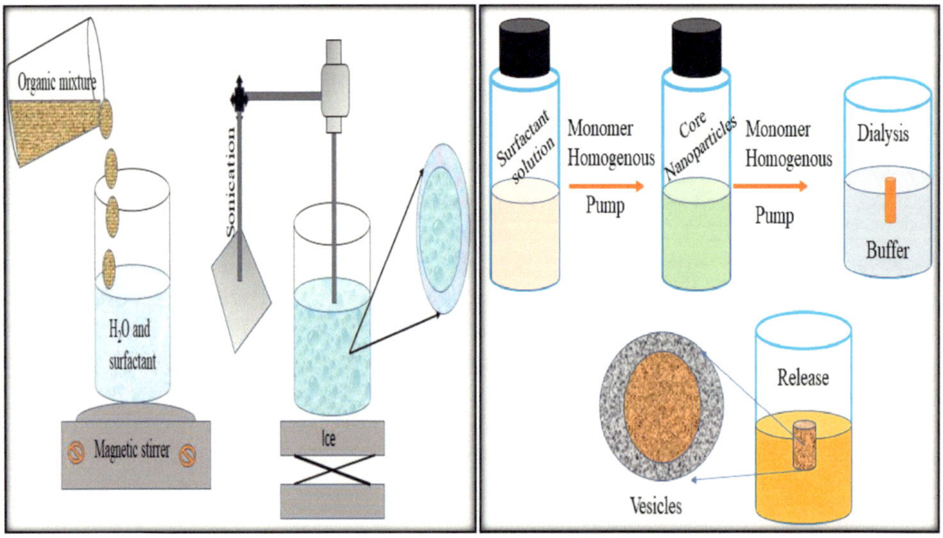

Figure 10.
Schematic diagrams representation of the advanced techniques for preparation of PNPs via sonication based system and csore- shell particulate system.

create different nano-particulate systems with different polymers, several techniques can be applied. The creation of multifunctional PNPs for single/dual or multiple drug release, including nano hydrogel, environment-responsive micelles, core-shell NPs, colloids, nano-spheres, and core-shell nano-spheres, has already been produced. The mechanism of the formulation approach is crucial in obtaining the required qualities. Therefore, having a synthesis technique available is crucial for approaching multi-functional PNPs with precise physiochemical characteristics for a given application.

Recent studies have focused on developing smart delivery methods for target biomolecules for a variety of therapies. The design of multi-functional PNPs for delivery of bioactives are closely related to the regulation of multiple cellular events. In particular, various peptides, proteins, growth factors, and cytokine therapy for different ailments are helpful in plying an important role in cellular responses [124]. In the sonication techniques, prob. sonication was used to generate the self-assembled NPs, and process involved cavitation, nucleation, and reversible locking concept, giving the formed nanostructure greater flexibility in its nature [125]. Self-assembled and core-shell particulate delivery systems, such as water-soluble polymeric drug compound conjugates, block polymeric micelles [126], long-circulating nano encapsulations, polymeric micelles, and core-shell nano-spheres were developed by using an in situ two-step semi-batch emulsion polymerization technique as a means of accurately and consistently delivering the right dose of drugs. Additionally, pH-responsive controlled release of hydrophobic anticancer drugs and its transport to tumor tissues/cells with acidic pH have been accomplished by core-shell nanospheres. Recently, an electrodropping system was designed and developed to create uniform, biocompatible core and shell capsules for angiogenesis in dual delivery systems [127], with an emphasis on regenerative medicine. The particle aggregation and drug encapsulation efficiency can be overcome by this electro-dropping technique.

In terms of micro-fluidics, the many applications have been significantly impacted by the cutting-edge science and technology used to manipulate micro/nano-scale volumes in micro-fluidic channels. Most micro-fluidic systems for synthesis, PNPs are still under development and they have the widest possible to develop because they are easily modifiable, highly reproducible, and can be combined with other techniques. Some advancement in micro-fluidics are anticipated to improve the preparation of PNPs and shift to clinical evaluation. Numerous microfluidic devices have recently been developed to allow quick mixing without the need of stimuli like electric force or stirring. The flow-focusing, droplet mixers, and other technologies are often used and enable micro-mixing inside the micro channel [128]. A fast solvent exchange through diffusion occurs as a result of the flow concentrating, which squeezes the solvent stream between two anti-solvent streams.

5. Future perspectives

The developments of the natural based PNPs have made the treatments to be more efficient and safe, utilizing the enormous variety of NPs design along with various functionalization. PNPs have to be biodegradable in nature and must possess a high capacity of circulation to avoid their removal from the systemic circulation. They developed systems should be nontoxic and non-immunogenic and should be able to produce the required effects as aimed. The role of copolymers could not be avoided in considering the tuning of the NPs system with the body components like blood proteins or mucosa which help in controlling their in vivo fate and the stabilizing of NPs.

Stimuli responding polymers are gaining interest for the coming future and research will be focused while considering their tuning properties for the development of NPs. The development of NPs with numerous potential, such as image contrast enhancement and targeting (as multifunctional NPs) has to be considered to match the various objectives required for the preparation and reaching hope of better scenario.

6. Conclusions

Natural polymers have been now taken into consideration for the development of NPs and are gaining sky-scraping consideration due to the biodegradability, biocompatibility, and flexibility ability of these materials using varieties of natural materials to obtain the required characteristics for a precise function. The continue demand for natural biomaterials has always been their due various advantages associated with these natural materials, like polysaccharides and proteins leading to the development of more stable formulation under industrial processing environment and biological matrix, through techniques such as cross-linking is among the most advanced research area nowadays while using different techniques.

Disclosures

There is no conflict of interest and disclosures associated with the manuscript.

Abbreviations

5-ALA	5-Aminolevulinic acid
BBB	Blood brain barrier.
CNCs	Cellulose nanocrystals.
DOX	Doxorubicin.
EDTA	ethylenediaminetetraacetic acid.
ESD	Emulsification/solvent diffusion.
HA	Hyaluronic acid.
HPMC	Hydroxy propyl methyl cellulose.
LDL	Low density lipoprotein.
MRSA	Methicillin resistant *S. aureus*.
NPs	Nanoparticles.
PNPs	Polymeric NPs.
PVA	Polyvinyl alcohol.
RES	Reticulo-endothelial system.
SF	Silk Fibroin.

Author details

Vikas Pandey[1*], Tanweer Haider[2], Poornima Agrawal[2], Sakshi Soni[2]
and Vandana Soni[2]

1 Amity Institute of Pharmacy, Amity University Gwalior, Madhya Pradesh, India

2 Department of Pharmaceutical Sciences, Dr. Harisingh Gour University, Sagar, India

*Address all correspondence to: vikaspandeydops@gmail.com
and vpandey@gwa.amity.edu

References

[1] Sung YK, Kim SW. Recent advances in polymeric drug delivery systems. Biomaterials Research. Dec 2020;**24**(1):1-12

[2] Bhushan B, Khanadeev V, Khlebtsov B, Khlebtsov N, Gopinath P. Impact of albumin based approaches in nanomedicine: Imaging, targeting and drug delivery. Advances in Colloid and Interface Science. 1 Aug 2017;**246**:13-39

[3] ud Din F, Aman W, Ullah I, Qureshi OS, Mustapha O, Shafique S, et al. Effective use of nanocarriers as drug delivery systems for the treatment of selected tumors. International Journal of Nanomedicine. 2017;**12**:7291

[4] Tong X, Pan W, Su T, Zhang M, Dong W, Qi X. Recent advances in natural polymer-based drug delivery systems. Reactive and Functional Polymers. 1 Mar 2020;**148**:104501

[5] Foox M, Zilberman M. Drug delivery from gelatin-based systems. Expert Opinion on Drug Delivery. 2015;**12**(9):1547-1563

[6] Alipal J, Pu'ad NM, Lee T, Nayan N, Sahari N, Basri H, et al. A review of gelatin: Properties, sources, process, applications, and commercialisation. Materials Today: Proceedings. 2021;**42**:240-250

[7] Mañes S, Llorente M, Lacalle RA, Gómez-Moutón C, Kremer L, Mira E, et al. The matrix metalloproteinase-9 regulates the insulin-like growth factor-triggered autocrine response in DU-145 carcinoma cells. Journal of Biological Chemistry. 1999;**274**(11):6935-6945

[8] Sahoo N, Sahoo RK, Biswas N, Guha A, Kuotsu K. Recent advancement of gelatin nanoparticles in drug and vaccine delivery. International Journal of Biological Macromolecules. 2015;**81**:317-331

[9] Saber MM. Strategies for surface modification of gelatin-based nanoparticles. Colloids and Surfaces B: Biointerfaces. 2019;**183**:110407

[10] Madkhali O, Mekhail G, Wettig SD. Modified gelatin nanoparticles for gene delivery. International Journal of Pharmaceutics. 2019;**554**:224-234

[11] Xu Y, Zhang J, Liu X, Huo P, Zhang Y, Chen H, et al. MMP-2-responsive gelatin nanoparticles for synergistic tumor therapy. Pharmaceutical Development and Technology. 2019;**24**(8):1002-1013

[12] Kirar S, Thakur NS, Laha JK, Bhaumik J, Banerjee UC. Development of gelatin nanoparticle-based biodegradable phototheranostic agents: advanced system to treat infectious diseases. ACS Biomaterials Science and Engineering. 2018;**4**(2):473-482

[13] Spada A, Emami J, Tuszynski JA, Lavasanifar A. The uniqueness of albumin as a carrier in nanodrug delivery. Molecular Pharmaceutics. 2021;**18**(5):1862-1894

[14] Karimi M, Bahrami S, Ravari SB, Zangabad PS, Mirshekari H, Bozorgomid M, et al. Albumin nanostructures as advanced drug delivery systems. Expert Opinion on Drug Delivery. 2016;**13**(11):1609-1623

[15] Tan YL, Ho HK. Navigating albumin-based nanoparticles through various drug delivery routes. Drug Discovery Today. 2018;**23**(5):1108-1114

[16] An F-F, Zhang X-H. Strategies for preparing albumin-based nanoparticles

for multifunctional bioimaging and drug delivery. Theranostics. 2017;7(15):3667

[17] Saleh T, Soudi T, Shojaosadati SA. Aptamer functionalized curcumin-loaded human serum albumin (HSA) nanoparticles for targeted delivery to HER-2 positive breast cancer cells. International Journal of Biological Macromolecules. 2019;**130**:109-116

[18] Xu L, He X-Y, Liu B-Y, Xu C, Ai S-L, Zhuo R-X, et al. Aptamer-functionalized albumin-based nanoparticles for targeted drug delivery. Colloids and Surfaces B: Biointerfaces. 2018;**171**:24-30

[19] Yu Z, Li X, Duan J, Yang X-D. Targeted treatment of colon cancer with aptamer-guided albumin nanoparticles loaded with docetaxel. International Journal of Nanomedicine. 2020;**15**:6737

[20] Zheng Y, Xie Q, Wang H, Hu Y, Ren B, Li X. Recent advances in plant polysaccharidemediated nano drug delivery systems. International Journal of Biological Macromolecules. 15 Dec 2020;**165**:2668-2683

[21] Iwao Y, Tomiguchi I, Domura A, Mantaira Y, Minami A, Suzuki T, et al. Inflamed site-specific drug delivery system based on the interaction of human serum albumin nanoparticles with myeloperoxidase in a murine model of experimental colitis. European Journal of Pharmaceutics and Biopharmaceutics: Official Journal of Arbeitsgemeinschaft fur Pharmazeutische Verfahrenstechnik. 2018;**125**:141-147

[22] Azevedo C, Nilsen J, Grevys A, Nunes R, Andersen JT, Sarmento BJ. Engineered albumin-functionalized nanoparticles for improved FcRn binding enhance oral delivery of insulin. The Journal of Controlled Release. 2020;**327**:161-173

[23] Karami E, Behdani M, Kazemi-Lomedasht F. Albumin nanoparticles as nanocarriers for drug delivery: Focusing on antibody and nanobody delivery and albumin-based drugs. Journal of Drug Delivery Science and Technology. 2020;**55**:101471

[24] Xenaki KT, Dorresteijn B, Muns JA, Adamzek K, Doulkeridou S, Houthoff H, et al. Homogeneous tumor targeting with a single dose of HER2-targeted albumin-binding domain-fused nanobody-drug conjugates results in long-lasting tumor remission in mice. Theranostics. 2021;**11**(11):5525

[25] Luo Z, Dai Y, Gao H. Development and application of hyaluronic acid in tumor targeting drug delivery. Acta Pharmaceutica Sinica B. 2019;**9**(6):1099-1112

[26] Huang G, Chen J. Preparation and applications of hyaluronic acid and its derivatives, International Journal of Biological Macromolecules. 2019;**125**:478-484

[27] Bai Y, Liu C-P, Chen D, Liu C-F, Zhuo L-H, Li H, et al. β-Cyclodextrin-modified hyaluronic acid-based supramolecular self-assemblies for pH-and esterase-dual-responsive drug delivery. Carbohydrate Polymers. 2020;**246**:116654

[28] Lu C, Xiao Y, Liu Y, Sun F, Qiu Y, Mu H, et al. Hyaluronic acid-based levofloxacin nanomicelles for nitric oxide-triggered drug delivery to treat bacterial infections. Carbohydrate Polymers. 2020;**229**:115479

[29] Duan Q, Ma L, Zhang B, Zhang Y, Li X, Wang T, et al. Construction and application of targeted drug delivery system based on hyaluronic acid and heparin functionalised carbon dots. Colloids and Surfaces B: Biointerfaces. 2020;**188**:110768

[30] Batool A, Arshad R, Razzaq S, Nousheen K, Kiani MH, Shahnaz G.

Formulation and evaluation of hyaluronic acid-based mucoadhesive self nanoemulsifying drug delivery system (SNEDDS) of tamoxifen for targeting breast cancer. International Journal of Biological Macromolecules. 2020;**152**:503-515

[31] Wani SUD, Gautam SP, Qadrie ZL, Gangadharappa HV. Silk fibroin as a natural polymeric based bio-material for tissue engineering and drug delivery systems—A review. International Journal of Biological Macromolecules. 2020;**163**:2145-2161

[32] Mottaghitalab F, Farokhi M, Shokrgozar MA, Atyabi F, Hosseinkhani H. Silk fibroin nanoparticle as a novel drug delivery system. The Journal of Controlled Release. 2015;**206**:161-176

[33] Tomeh MA, Hadianamrei R, Zhao X. Silk fibroin as a functional biomaterial for drug and gene delivery. Pharmaceutics. 2019;**11**(10):494

[34] Pandey V, Haider T, Jain P, Gupta PN, Soni V. Silk as a leading-edge biological macromolecule for improved drug delivery. Journal of Drug Delivery Science and Technology. 1 Feb 2020;**55**:101294

[35] Cao Y, Liu F, Chen Y, Yu T, Lou D, Guo Y, et al. Drug release from core-shell PVA/silk fibroin nanoparticles fabricated by one-step electrospraying. Scientific Reports. 2017;**7**(1):1-9

[36] Chouhan D, Mandal BB. Silk biomaterials in wound healing and skin regeneration therapeutics: From bench to bedside. Acta Biomaterialia. 2020;**103**:24-51

[37] Gangrade A, Mandal BB. Injectable carbon nanotube impregnated silk based multifunctional hydrogel for localized targeted and on-demand anticancer drug delivery. ACS Biomaterials Science & Engineering. 2019;**5**(5):2365-2381

[38] Gough CR, Hu X. Air-spun silk-based micro-/nanofibers and thin films for drug delivery. International Journal of Molecular Sciences. 2021;**22**(17):9588

[39] Zhang H, Liu Y, Chen C, Cui W, Zhang C, Ye F, et al. Responsive drug-delivery microcarriers based on the silk fibroin inverse opal scaffolds for controllable drug release. Applied Materials Today. 2020;**19**:100540

[40] Hu J, Albadawi H, Zhang Z, Salomao MA, Gunduz S, Rehman S, et al. Silk embolic material for catheter-directed endovascular drug delivery. Advanced Materials. 2022;**34**(2):2106865

[41] Sun B, Zhang M, Shen J, He Z, Fatehi P, Ni Y. Applications of cellulose-based materials in sustained drug delivery systems. Current Medicinal Chemistry. 2019;**26**(14):2485-2501

[42] Gupta B, Mishra V, Gharat S, Momin M, Omri A. Cellulosic polymers for enhancing drug bioavailability in ocular drug delivery systems. Pharmaceuticals (Basel). 2021;**14**(11):1201

[43] Sheng Y, Gao J, Yin Z-Z, Kang J, Kong Y. Dual-drug delivery system based on the hydrogels of alginate and sodium carboxymethyl cellulose for colorectal cancer treatment. Carbohydrate Polymers. 2021;**269**:118325

[44] Pooresmaeil M, Nia SB, Namazi H. Green encapsulation of LDH (Zn/Al)-5-Fu with carboxymethyl cellulose biopolymer; new nanovehicle for oral colorectal cancer treatment. International Journal of Biological Macromolecules. 2019;**139**:994-1001

[45] Troncoso OP, Torres FG. Non-conventional starch nanoparticles for drug delivery applications. Medical Devices & Sensors. 2020;**3**(6):e10111

[46] Shehabeldine A, Hasanin M. Green synthesis of hydrolyzed starch–chitosan nano-composite as drug delivery system to gram negative bacteria. Environmental Nanotechnology, Monitoring & Management. 2019;**12**:100252

[47] Grigoras AG. Drug delivery systems using pullulan, a biocompatible polysaccharide produced by fungal fermentation of starch. Environmental Chemistry Letters. 2019;**17**(3):1209-1223

[48] Nallasamy P, Ramalingam T, Nooruddin T, Shanmuganathan R, Arivalagan P, Natarajan S. Polyherbal drug loaded starch nanoparticles as promising drug delivery system: Antimicrobial, antibiofilm and neuroprotective studies. Process Biochemistry. 2020;**92**:355-364

[49] Utsumi S, Matsumura Y. Structure-function relationships. Food proteins and their Applications. 1997;**80**:257

[50] Chua J-Y, Liu S-Q. Soy whey: More than just wastewater from tofu and soy protein isolate industry. Trends in Food Science & Technology. 2019;**91**:24-32

[51] Tansaz S, Boccaccini AR. Biomedical applications of soy protein: A brief overview. Journal of Biomedical Materials Research Part A. 2016;**104**(2): 553-569

[52] Yu Z, Sun L, Wang W, Zeng W, Mustapha A, Lin M. Soy protein-based films incorporated with cellulose nanocrystals and pine needle extract for active packaging. Industrial Crops and Products. 2018;**112**:412-419

[53] Cheng X, Zeng X, Li D, Wang X, Sun M, He L, et al. TPGS-grafted and acid-responsive soy protein nanogels for efficient intracellular drug release, accumulation, penetration in 3D tumor spheroids of drug-resistant cancer cells. Materials Science and Engineering: C. 2019;**102**:863-875

[54] Zheng Z, Olayinka O, Li B. 2S-soy protein-based biopolymer as a non-covalent surfactant and its effects on electrical conduction and dielectric relaxation of polymer nanocomposites. Engineered Science. 2018;**4**(18):87-99

[55] Luo X, Liu J, Zheng P, Li M, Zhou Y, Huang L, et al. Promoting enzymatic hydrolysis of lignocellulosic biomass by inexpensive soy protein. Biotechnology for Biofuels. 2019;**12**(1):1-13

[56] Phuhongsung P, Zhang M, Bhandari B. 4D printing of products based on soy protein isolate via microwave heating for flavor development. Food Research International. 2020;**137**:109605

[57] De Marco I. Zein microparticles and nanoparticles as drug delivery systems. Polymers. 2022;**14**(11):2172

[58] Raza A, Hayat U, Bilal M, Iqbal HM, Wang J-Y. Zein-based micro-and nano-constructs and biologically therapeutic cues with multi-functionalities for oral drug delivery systems. Journal of Drug Delivery Science and Technology. 2020;**58**:101818

[59] Reboredo C, González-Navarro C, Martínez-Oharriz C, Martínez-López A, Irache J. Preparation and evaluation of PEG-coated zein nanoparticles for oral drug delivery purposes. International Journal of Pharmaceutics. 2021;**597**:120287

[60] Yurdasiper A, Sevgi F. An overview of modified release chitosan, alginate and eudragit RS microparticles. Journal of Chemical and Pharmaceutical Research. 2010;**2**(3):704-721

[61] Santinon C, Borges D, da Silva MGC, Vieira MGA. Evaluation of different covalent crosslinking agents into

valsartan-loaded sericin and alginate particles for modified release. Powder Technology. 2021;**390**:240-255

[62] Jahanban-Esfahlan R, Derakhshankhah H, Haghshenas B, Massoumi B, Abbasian M, Jaymand M. A bio-inspired magnetic natural hydrogel containing gelatin and alginate as a drug delivery system for cancer chemotherapy. International Journal of Biological Macromolecules. 2020;**156**:438-445

[63] Tønnesen HH, Karlsen J. Alginate in drug delivery systems. Drug Development and Industrial Pharmacy. 2002;**28**(6):621-630

[64] Qureshi D, Nayak SK, Maji S, Kim D, Banerjee I, Pal K. Carrageenan: A wonder polymer from marine algae for potential drug delivery applications. Current Pharmaceutical Design. 2019;**25**(11):1172-1186

[65] Shah ZC, Huffman FG. Current availability and consumption of carrageenan-containing foods. Ecology of Food and Nutrition. 2003;**42**(6):357-371

[66] Khan MUA, Raza MA, Mehboob H, Kadir MRA, Abd Razak SI, Shah SA, et al. Development and in vitro evaluation of κ-carrageenan based polymeric hybrid nanocomposite scaffolds for bone tissue engineering. RSC Advances. 2020;**10**(66):40529-40542

[67] Vijayakumar S, Saravanakumar K, Malaikozhundan B, Divya M, Vaseeharan B, Durán-Lara EF, et al. Biopolymer K-carrageenan wrapped ZnO nanoparticles as drug delivery vehicles for anti MRSA therapy. International Journal of Biological Macromolecules. 2020;**144**:9-18

[68] Oliyaei N, Moosavi-Nasab M, Mazloomi SM. Therapeutic activity of fucoidan and carrageenan as marine algal polysaccharides against viruses. 3 Biotech. 2022;**12**(7):1-15

[69] Bernkop-Schnürch A, Dünnhaupt S. Chitosan-based drug delivery systems. European Journal of Pharmaceutics and Biopharmaceutics. 2012;**81**(3):463-469

[70] Wang W, Meng Q, Li Q, Liu J, Zhou M, Jin Z, et al. Chitosan derivatives and their application in biomedicine. International Journal of Molecular Sciences. 2020;**21**(2):487

[71] Baghaei M, Tekie FSM, Khoshayand MR, Varshochian R, Hajiramezanali M, Kachousangi MJ, et al. Optimization of chitosan-based polyelectrolyte nanoparticles for gene delivery, using design of experiment: In vitro and in vivo study. Materials Science & Engineering C-Materials for Biological Applications. 2021;**118**:111036

[72] Ziminska M, Wilson JJ, McErlean E, Dunne N, McCarthy H. Synthesis and evaluation of a thermoresponsive degradable chitosan-grafted PNIPAAm hydrogel as a "smart" gene delivery system. Materials (Basel). 2020;**13**(11):2530

[73] de Jesus Raposo MF, De Morais AMB, De Morais RMSC. Marine polysaccharides from algae with potential biomedical applications. Marine Drugs. 2015;**13**(5):2967-3028

[74] Zhong H, Gao X, Cheng C, Liu C, Wang Q, Han X. The structural characteristics of seaweed polysaccharides and their application in gel drug delivery systems. Marine Drugs. 2020;**18**(12):658

[75] Lu K-Y, Li R, Hsu C-H, Lin C-W, Chou S-C, Tsai M-L, et al. Development of a new type of multifunctional fucoidan-based nanoparticles for anticancer drug delivery. Carbohydrate Polymers. 2017;**165**:410-420

[76] Sezer AD, Cevher E. Fucoidan: A versatile biopolymer for biomedical applications. Active Implants and Scaffolds for Tissue Regeneration. 2011:377-406

[77] Choi J-i, Kim H-J. Preparation of low molecular weight fucoidan by gamma-irradiation and its anticancer activity. Carbohydrate Polymers. 2013;**97**(2):358-362

[78] Shanmugapriya K, Kang HW. Synthesis of nanohydroxyapatite/collagen-loaded fucoidan-based composite hydrogel for drug delivery to gastrointestinal cancer cells. Colloids and Surfaces B: Biointerfaces. 2021;**203**:111769

[79] Calzoni E, Cesaretti A, Polchi A, Di Michele A, Tancini B, Emiliani C. Biocompatible polymer nanoparticles for drug delivery applications in cancer and neurodegenerative disorder therapies. Journal of Functional Biomaterials. 2019;**10**(1):4

[80] Tran S, DeGiovanni P-J, Piel B, Rai P. Cancer nanomedicine: A review of recent success in drug delivery. Clinical and Translational Medicine. 2017;**6**(1):1-21

[81] Bregoli L, Movia D, Gavigan-Imedio JD, Lysaght J, Reynolds J, Prina-Mello A. Nanomedicine applied to translational oncology: A future perspective on cancer treatment. Nanomedicine. 2016;**12**(1):81-103

[82] Ahmad N, Ahmad R, Alam MA, Ahmad FJ. Enhancement of oral bioavailability of doxorubicin through surface modified biodegradable polymeric nanoparticles. Chemistry Central Journal. 2018;**12**(1):1-14

[83] Soma CE, Dubernet C, Bentolila D, Benita S, Couvreur P. Reversion of multidrug resistance by co-encapsulation of doxorubicin and cyclosporin A in polyalkylcyanoacrylate nanoparticles. Biomaterials. 2000;**21**(1):1-7

[84] Zhao Y, Cai C, Liu M, Zhao Y, Pei W, Chu X, et al. An organic solvent-free technology for the fabrication of albumin-based paclitaxel nanoparticles for effective cancer therapy. Colloids and Surfaces B: Biointerfaces. 2019;**183**:110394

[85] Çırpanlı Y, Allard E, Passirani C, Bilensoy E, Lemaire L, Çalış S, et al. Antitumoral activity of camptothecin-loaded nanoparticles in 9L rat glioma model. The International Journal of Pharmaceutics. 2011;**403**(1-2):201-206

[86] Khanna V, Kalscheuer S, Kirtane A, Zhang W, Panyam J. Perlecan-targeted nanoparticles for drug delivery to triple-negative breast cancer. Future Drug Discovery. 2019;**1**(1):FDD8

[87] Hu D, Chen L, Qu Y, Peng J, Chu B, Shi K, et al. Oxygen-generating hybrid polymeric nanoparticles with encapsulated doxorubicin and chlorin e6 for trimodal imaging-guided combined chemo-photodynamic therapy. Theranostics. 2018;**8**(6):1558

[88] Zhu D, Tao W, Zhang H, Liu G, Wang T, Zhang L, et al. Docetaxel (DTX)-loaded polydopamine-modified TPGS-PLA nanoparticles as a targeted drug delivery system for the treatment of liver cancer. Acta Biomaterialia. 2016;**30**:144-154

[89] Guo J, Gao X, Su L, Xia H, Gu G, Pang Z, et al. Aptamer-functionalized PEG–PLGA nanoparticles for enhanced anti-glioma drug delivery. Biomaterials. 2011;**32**(31):8010-8020

[90] Shafiei-Irannejad V, Samadi N, Salehi R, Yousefi B, Rahimi M, Akbarzadeh A, et al. Reversion of multidrug resistance by co-encapsulation of doxorubicin and metformin in poly (lactide-co-glycolide)-d-α-tocopheryl polyethylene glycol 1000 succinate

nanoparticles. Pharmaceutical Research. 2018;**35**(6):1-13

[91] Jin M, Jin G, Kang L, Chen L, Gao Z, Huang W. Smart polymeric nanoparticles with pH-responsive and PEG-detachable properties for co-delivering paclitaxel and survivin siRNA to enhance antitumor outcomes. The International Journal of Nanomedicine. 2018;**13**:2405

[92] Rao JP, Geckeler KE. Polymer nanoparticles: Preparation techniques and size-control parameters. Progress in Polymer Science. 2011;**36**(7):887-913

[93] Reis CP, Neufeld RJ, Ribeiro AJ, Veiga F. Nanoencapsulation I. Methods for preparation of drug-loaded polymeric nanoparticles. Nanomedicine. 2006;**2**(1):8-21

[94] Fessi H, Puisieux F, Devissaguet JP, Ammoury N, Benita S. Nanocapsule formation by interfacial polymer deposition following solvent displacement. International Journal of Pharmaceutics. 1989;**55**(1):R1-R4

[95] Barichello JM, Morishita M, Takayama K, Nagai T. Encapsulation of hydrophilic and lipophilic drugs in PLGA nanoparticles by the nanoprecipitation method. Drug Development and Industrial Pharmacy. 1999;**25**(4):471-476

[96] Quintanar-Guerrero D, Allémann E, Fessi H, Doelker E. Preparation techniques and mechanisms of formation of biodegradable nanoparticles from preformed polymers. Drug Development and Industrial Pharmacy. 1998;**24**(12):1113-1128

[97] Vauthier C, Dubernet C, Fattal E, Pinto-Alphandary H, Couvreur P. Poly (alkylcyanoacrylates) as biodegradable materials for biomedical applications. Advanced Drug Delivery Reviews. 2003;**55**(4):519-548

[98] Wehrle P, Magenheim B, Benita S. The influence of process parameters on the PLA nanoparticle size distribution, evaluated by means of factorial design. European Journal of Pharmaceutics and Biopharmaceutics. 1995;**41**(1):19-26

[99] Arbós P, Wirth M, Arangoa M, Gabor F, Irache JM. Gantrez® AN as a new polymer for the preparation of ligand–nanoparticle conjugates. The Journal of Controlled Release. 2002;**83**(3):321-330

[100] Irache JM, Huici M, Konecny M, Espuelas S, Campanero MA, Arbos P. Bioadhesive properties of Gantrez nanoparticles. Molecules. 2005;**10**(1):126-145

[101] Prasad R, Pandey R, Varma A, Barman I. Polymer based nanoparticles for drug delivery systems and cancer therapeutics. Natural Polymers for Drug Delivery. 2016:53-70

[102] Memişoğlu E, Bochot A, Özalp M, Şen M, Duchêne D, Hincal A. Direct formation of nanospheres from amphiphilic β-cyclodextrin inclusion complexes. Pharmaceutical Research. 2003;**20**(1):117-125

[103] Sun Y, Wang J, Zhang X, Zhang Z, Zheng Y, Chen D, et al. Synchronic release of two hormonal contraceptives for about one month from the PLGA microspheres: In vitro and in vivo studies. The Journal of Controlled Release. 2008;**129**(3):192-199

[104] El-Shabouri MH. Positively charged nanoparticles for improving the oral bioavailability of cyclosporin-A. The International Journal of Pharmaceutics. 2002;**249**(1-2):101-108

[105] Jung T, Kamm W, Breitenbach A, Kaiserling E, Xiao J, Kissel TJE. Biodegradable nanoparticles for oral

delivery of peptides: is there a role for polymers to affect mucosal uptake? European Journal of Pharmaceutics and Biopharmaceutics. 2000;**50**(1):147-160

[106] Nagavarma B, Yadav HK, Ayaz A, Vasudha L, Shivakumar HG. Different techniques for preparation of polymeric nanoparticles—A review. Asian Journal of Pharmaceutical and Clinical Research. 2012;**5**(3):16-23

[107] Jeon H-J, Jeong Y-I, Jang M-K, Park Y-H, Nah J-W. Effect of solvent on the preparation of surfactant-free poly (DL-lactide-co-glycolide) nanoparticles and norfloxacin release characteristics. The International Journal of Pharmaceutics. 2000;**207**(1-2):99-108

[108] Jeong YI, Cho CS, Kim SH, Ko KS, Kim SI, Shim YH, et al. Preparation of poly (DL-lactide-co-glycolide) nanoparticles without surfactant. Journal of Applied Polymer Science. 2001;**80**(12):2228-2236

[109] Kostag M, Köhler S, Liebert T, Heinze T. Pure cellulose nanoparticles from trimethylsilyl cellulose. Paper Presented at the Macromolecular Symposia. 2010;**294**(2):96-106

[110] Chronopoulou L, Fratoddi I, Palocci C, Venditti I, Russo MV. Osmosis based method drives the self-assembly of polymeric chains into micro- and nanostructures. Langmuir. 2009;**25**(19):11940-11946

[111] York P. Strategies for particle design using supercritical fluid technologies. Pharmaceutical Science & Technology Today. 1999;**2**(11):430-440

[112] Blasig A, Shi C, Enick RM, Thies M. Effect of concentration and degree of saturation on RESS of a CO_2-soluble fluoropolymer. Industrial and Engineering Chemistry Research. 2002;**41**(20):4976-4983

[113] Chernyak Y, Henon F, Harris RB, Gould RD, Franklin RK, Edwards JR, et al. Formation of perfluoropolyether coatings by the rapid expansion of supercritical solutions (RESS) process. Part 1: Experimental results. Industrial & Engineering Chemistry Research. 2001;**40**(26):6118-6126

[114] Meziani MJ, Pathak P, Wang W, Desai T, Patil A, Sun Y-P. Polymeric nanofibers from rapid expansion of supercritical solution. Industrial & Engineering Chemistry Research. 2005;**44**(13):4594-4598

[115] Lowe PJ, Temple CS. Calcitonin and insulin in isobutylcyanoacrylate nanocapsules: protection against proteases and effect on intestinal absorption in rats. Journal of Pharmacy and Pharmacology. 1994;**46**(7):547-552

[116] Kreuter J. On the mechanism of termination in heterogeneous polymerization. Journal of Polymer Science: Polymer Letters Edition. 1982;**20**(10):543-545

[117] Puig JE. Microemulsion polymerization. Polymeric Materials Encyclopedia. 1996;**6**:4333-4341

[118] Scott C, Wu D, Ho C-C, Co CC. Liquid-core capsules via interfacial polymerization: A free-radical analogy of the nylon rope trick. Journal of the American Chemical Society. 2005;**127**(12):4160-4161

[119] Gallardo M, Couarraze G, Denizot B, Treupel L, Couvreur P, Puisieux F. Study of the mechanisms of formation of nanoparticles and nanocapsules of polyisobutyl-2-cyanoacrylate. International Journal of Pharmaceutics. 1993;**100**(1-3):55-64

[120] Braunecker WA, Matyjaszewski K. Controlled/living radical polymerization:

Features, developments, and perspectives. Progress in Polymer Science. 2007;**32**(1):93-146

[121] Dustgania A, Vasheghani Farahani E, Imani M. Preparation of chitosan nanoparticles loaded by dexamethasone sodium phosphate. Iranian Journal of Pharmaceutical Sciences. 2008;**4**(2):111-114

[122] Nuxoll E. BioMEMS in drug delivery. Advanced Drug Delivery Reviews. 2013;**65**(11-12):1611-1625

[123] Wang Y, Byrne JD, Napier ME, DeSimone JM. Engineering nanomedicines using stimuli-responsive biomaterials. Advanced Drug Delivery Reviews. 2012;**64**(11):1021-1030

[124] Kronenberg HM. Developmental regulation of the growth plate. Nature. 2003;**423**(6937):332-336

[125] Marimuthu M, Bennet D, Kim S. Self-assembled nanoparticles of PLGA-conjugated glucosamine as a sustained transdermal drug delivery vehicle. Polymer Journal. 2013;**45**(2):202-209

[126] Kopeček J, Kopečková P, Minko T, Lu Z-R, Peterson CM. Water soluble polymers in tumor targeted delivery. The Journal of Controlled Release. 2001;**74**(1-3):147-158

[127] Valencia PM, Farokhzad OC, Karnik R, Langer R. Microfluidic technologies for accelerating the clinical translation of nanoparticles. Nature Nanotechnology. 2020:93-112

[128] Valencia PM, Basto PA, Zhang L, Rhee M, Langer R, Farokhzad OC, et al. Single-step assembly of homogenous lipid–polymeric and lipid–quantum dot nanoparticles enabled by microfluidic rapid mixing. ACS Nano. 2010;**4**(3):1671-1679

Chapter 3

Recent Strategies for Ocular Drug Delivery: Promises and Challenges

Amal H. El-Kamel and Asmaa A. Ashour

Abstract

Ocular diseases include various anterior and posterior segment diseases. Due to the unique anatomy and physiology of the eye, efficient ocular drug delivery is a great challenge to researchers. The emerging nanoscience is playing an important role in the development of novel strategies for ocular disease management. Various active molecules have been designed to associate with nanocarriers to overcome ocular barriers and interact with certain ocular tissues. In this chapter, highlights will be made on barrier to intraocular delivery, general pathways for ocular absorption, and factors affecting intraocular bioavailability. The recent attempts of nanotechnology for treating anterior and posterior ocular diseases will be explored. This will include nanomicelles, nanoparticles, nanosuspensions, vesicular systems, in situ gel, dendrimers, contact lenses, implants, microneedles, and cell-based delivery systems. In addition, gene-based ocular delivery systems will be discussed. In this chapter, we will also provide a comprehensive overview of drug-device combinations used for ocular diseases such as glaucoma, dry eye disease, infections, and inflammations. Furthermore, drug delivery devices for ocular surgeries are discussed. Finally, challenges and future prospective of ocular delivery systems will be explored.

Keywords: nanocarriers, microneedles, gene, cell-based therapy, ocular devices

1. Introduction

Globally, eye diseases and consequential visual impairment are considered as the nation's absolute threat, compromising physical and mental health. As reported by the World Health Organization, worldwide, the number of people suffering from visual impairment is more than 2.2 billion [1]. Additionally, an analysis by Lancet Glob Health stated that, as population gets older, the number of moderate to severe vision impairment and blindness cases would increase to 600 million and 115 million by 2050, respectively [1].

Anatomically speaking, the human eye consists of two regions: the anterior segment including aqueous humor, cornea, conjunctiva, iris, ciliary body, and lens. Whereas the posterior segment includes vitreous humor, retina, choroid, and optic nerve. In other words, the eye consists of several attached tissue layers. In the anterior segment, the collagenous layer providing the mechanical strength is the cornea that is responsible for focusing the light on the retina. In the posterior segment, the opaque collagenous layer is the fibrous sclera. The middle layer in the anterior segment is called Uvea, which involves the iris and ciliary body. The ciliary body contains smooth muscles that produce the aqueous humor. The latter has many functions such as suppling nutrients to the avascular tissues in the anterior segment, maintaining the intraocular pressure, and drainage of waste from lens and cornea. In the posterior segment, the middle layer comprises enormous network of capillaries called vascular choroid that provides the retina with all the essential nutrients. The innermost layer is the retina, which transports the light signal to the brain [2].

Based on the aforementioned background, the eye comprises unique anatomical and physiological barriers hindering effective intraocular drug delivery that would be discussed in the following section.

2. Barriers to intraocular drug delivery

The eye consists of numerous barriers and defense mechanisms to protect it from the environment. Barriers to intraocular drug delivery are categorized as physiological and anatomical. Physiological barriers involve blinking, tear turn over and naso-lachrymal drainage. Whereas anatomical barriers include various static and dynamic barriers that impede drug entry into the eye segment [3].

In the anterior chamber, the static barriers are corneal epithelium, stroma, and blood aqueous barrier (BAB). Whereas dynamic barriers are the conjunctival blood and lymph flow along with tear drainage. BAB consists of tight junctions between the non-pigmented epithelial cells in the ciliary body, junctions of the iridial tissues as well as the blood vessels of the iris. BAB restricts the movement of molecules from blood to aqueous humor through iris ciliary capillaries [3].

In the posterior chamber, static barriers are sclera, bruch's membrane in choroid, and blood retinal barrier (BRB), which involves tight junctions in retinal capillary endothelial cells and retinal pigmented epithelium. While dynamic barriers comprise the drainage of administered drugs by blood and lymphatic vessels [3].

It is worth mentioning that the blood ocular barrier consists of both BAB and BRB. Its function is to maintain optimum intraocular pressure via preserving the fluid composition of the eye [3].

Mucin, covering the corneal and conjunctival surfaces for protection, constitutes an additional ocular barrier for diffusion of large drugs molecules. Moreover, the expression of many efflux pumps (P-glycoprotein, multidrug-resistant protein, and breast cancer resistant protein) on the capillary endothelium represents another barrier limiting drug ocular bioavailability [3].

3. General pathways for ocular absorption

Absorption of drug into the inner eye occurs through two major pathways, either corneal or non-corneal. The corneal route is considered as the major pathway for ocular drug absorption after topical administration. This route involves the penetration of the administered drug through the corneal epithelium. Afterward, the drug gets to the corneal stroma, endothelium, and aqueous humor. Subsequently, the drug may either be eliminated by the drainage of the aqueous humor through trabecular meshwork into Schlemm's canal, or it may reach the iris-ciliary body blood vessels and then enter the systemic circulation. Additionally, drugs also may distribute to a lesser extent to the lens and vitreous humor from the aqueous humor [4].

On the other hand, the non-corneal route for ocular drug absorption encompasses the passage of drugs across the conjunctiva and sclera. After that, they reach the ciliary body followed by the iris without access to the aqueous humor. Concerning the non-corneal route, it is important to highlight that the conjunctiva contains numerous blood vessels. Accordingly, a large portion of the drug dose is suspected to enter the blood circulation rather than diffusing into the sclera [4].

The next section designates the different factors affecting intraocular drug bioavailability, which makes ocular delivery challenging.

4. Factors influencing intraocular drug bioavailability

Poor ocular bioavailability of the topically administered drugs represents a main concern associated with ophthalmic dosage forms. The presence of numerous physiological and anatomical constraints resulted in absorption of a very small portion of the topically instilled dose. The several factors affecting drug ocular bioavailability will be discussed in detail in the following subsections.

4.1 Precorneal fluid drainage

It constitutes one of the major reasons for poor ocular drug absorption. A large portion of the topically instilled volume (~80–90%) is drained into the nasolacrimal duct. The nasolacrimal drainage aids in preserving a fixed volume of the precorneal fluid (~7–10 μl). Consequently, it represents a natural protective physiological mechanism that is responsible for loss of any excess fluid.

The factors affecting the drainage rate include the Instilled volume, viscosity, pH, tonicity, and drug type. Concerning the instilled volume, the larger the volume, the more the drainage. For viscosity, increasing viscosity of an instilled dose results in prolongation of its ocular residence time. Regarding the pH effect, instillation of alkaline or acidic solutions gives rise to excessive lacrimation and hence loss of the administered medication. Therefore, the pH of the ophthalmic formulations must be adjusted to 7–7.7 to mimic the physiological pH of tear fluid (7.4). Regarding tonicity, preparations intended for ocular use should be isotonic with tear fluid. Severe irritation with excessive tear secretion occurs upon instillation of hypertonic solutions. As for drug type, it was reported that certain drugs can affect tear secretion. For instance, epinephrine can induce lacrimation, while tetracaine can suppress it [3].

4.2 Binding of drugs to tear proteins or melanin

The protein content of the tear fluid is ~0.7% of total body protein. Binding of drugs to tear proteins may bring about a significant decrease in drug concentration reaching the target site [3].

Concerning melanin binding, certain drugs such as ephedrine and timolol were reported to possess a high binding affinity to melanin pigment present in the iris and ciliary body, thereby lowering their ocular bioavailability [3].

4.3 Drug absorption to the systemic circulation

It may occur either directly from the conjunctival blood capillaries or after drainage of the instilled solution to the nasal cavity. Accordingly, this can result in remarkable drug loss into the systemic circulation, hence lowering its ocular bioavailability [3].

4.4 Corneal barrier

Cornea is a complex tissue that is made of six different layers. It plays an essential role in decreasing drug ocular bioavailability acting as a physical constraint impeding drug permeability [3].

4.5 Drug metabolism

Several metabolizing enzymes (cytochrome P450, cyclooxygenases, aldehyde oxidases, and monoamine oxidases) are expressed in various ocular tissues as cornea, lens, iris, ciliary body, and retina. These enzymes have the ability to metabolize the instilled drugs, decreasing their ocular bioavailability [3].

5. Nanocarriers for ocular drug delivery

As illustrated previously, drug delivery to the eye is challenging for formulators owing to its barrier nature. Additionally, the chronic nature of various ocular diseases necessitates frequent administration of drugs. In this context, nanocarriers are elaborated to overcome the limitations of conventional ocular formulations as well as guarantee controlled and targeted drug delivery [5].

Nano delivery systems are colloidal systems with a particle size in the nanometer range (10–1000 nm) and a certain surface charge. They have various biomedical applications depending on their size. Additionally, their surface charge contributes to their retention at the specific site. For example, the negative charge on the surface of both the corneal and conjunctival tissues paves the way for cationic nanoparticles to be interacted to these tissues via electrostatic attraction. Consequently, increasing their residence in the anterior segment of the eye [5].

Based on the aforementioned background, nanocarriers are predicted to overcome the numerous ocular barriers thanks to their unique nano-size and surface characteristics. The different nanocarriers and their targeting ability for ocular drug delivery will be presented in detail in the following subsections.

5.1 Nanomicelles

Nanomicelles are nanostructures (10–100 nm) formed spontaneously in the aqueous environment by the self-assembly of certain block copolymers having amphoteric properties. They have many advantages for ocular drug delivery such as enhancing the aqueous solubility and stability for the hydrophobic drugs, prolongation of drugs' ocular retention, improving drug corneal permeability, and modification of drug release [1]. The amphoteric nature of the nanomicelles facilitates their penetration through both lipophilic (corneal epithelial and endothelial cells) and hydrophilic matrices. As well, their small size permits their uptake by the corneal cells. Moreover, they were reported to improve drug bioavailability by inhibiting the efflux transporter proteins by the use of the proper surfactants in their backbone structure [1, 6].

Accordingly, nanomicelles have attracted increasing attention as noninvasive ocular drug delivery systems owing to their unique properties.

Concerning the targeting potential of the nanomicelles to the anterior segment of the eye, several studies have reported that the administration of the drug in a nanomicellar formulation rather than ointment, suspension, or emulsion formulations resulted in improved corneal, trans-corneal, and conjunctival uptake [7]. The clear Cyclosporine-A nanomicellar formulation prepared by Cholkar et al. [8] for treatment of dry eye disease in rabbits was approved by the United States Food and Drug Administration (FDA) in 2018. Cequa® (cyclosporine-A 0.09%) is a unique nanomicellar formulation, that is a clear solution approved for clinical use. In another study, Safwat et al. [9] prepared poly ethylene glycol-block-poly lactic acid nanomicelles containing triamcinolone acetonide. The selected formulations were dispersed into chitosan hydrogel to evaluate their anti-inflammatory potential in a carrageenan-induced ocular inflammatory rabbit model. The prepared micelles had good in-vitro characteristics (size: 176.80 ± 2.25 nm, drug loading: 15–25%, sustained drug release over a period of 1 week and 10-fold increase in drug aqueous solubility). Furthermore, the elaborated micellar hydrogel formulation resulted in complete disappearance of the corneal inflammatory signs in tested rabbits based on histopathological examination [9].

For targeting posterior segment of the eye, Xu et al. [10] prepared chitosan oligosaccharide-valylvaline-stearic acid nanomicelles to actively target peptide transporter-1 for topical ocular dexamethasone delivery to treat macular edema. Fluorescence microscopical images of frozen sections for various ocular tissues from tested animals indicated that the coumarin-6 labeled nanomicelles reached the posterior segment mainly through conjunctival route. Following topical administration, dexamethasone concentration in the posterior segment reached the therapeutic levels at 0.5 h and 1 h and can still be detected at 1.5 h post administration [10].

5.2 Polymeric nanoparticles

Polymeric nanoparticles made of biodegradable polymers and having sizes from 10 to 100 nm are widely used in ocular therapy. These nanocarriers consist of various polymers, in which the drug may be just adsorbed on the surface or incorporated into the polymer matrix. Polymeric nanoparticles offer numerous advantages for ocular delivery, which mainly related to their unique properties, as biodegradability, biocompatibility, and muco-adhesiveness. Therefore, pericorneal retention time is prolonged, and hence drug bioavailability is improved. For that purpose, many researchers prepared ocular drug delivery systems coated with mucoadhesive polymers (poloxamers, hyaluronic acid, chitosan, sodium alginate, among others) to increase drug ocular bioavailability [11].

For instance, Radwan et al. [12] prepared bovine serum albumin nanoparticles coated with chitosan by the desolvation method for the topical delivery of tetrandrine for management of glaucoma. The optimized formulation had a size of 237.9 nm and zeta potential of 24 mV and high % EE > 95% with a sustained-release drug profile. Moreover, the prepared nanosystem exhibited a significantly enhanced ex -vivo transcorneal permeation with improved in-vitro antioxidant and antiproliferative action on corneal stromal fibroblasts. In addition, the elaborated formulation succeeded to increase the drug bioavailability in the aqueous humor of treated rabbits by twofold compared with the free drug together with a remarkable reduction in intraocular pressure in a rabbit model for glaucoma.

In order to achieve active targeting to the posterior eye chamber for treatment of diabetic retinopathy, apatinib -loaded bovine serum albumin nanoparticles coated with hyaluronic acid were developed [13]. Hyaluronic acid was exploited to achieve a dual role as a mucoadhesive polymer with capability to target the CD44 receptors expressed on retinal cells. The elaborated nanoplatform had good colloidal and mucoadhesive properties with no in-vitro cytotoxicity on rabbit corneal epithelial cells. The in-vivo evaluation revealed the ability of the topically instilled nano formulation to alleviate the corneal histopathological manifestations in diabetic retinopathy rat model with improved retinal accumulation as evidenced by confocal microscopy [13].

5.3 Lipid-based nanoparticles

Solid lipid nanoparticles (SLNs) are nanocarrier systems (10–500 nm) consist of lipids dispersed in an aqueous surfactant system. They are reserved for the delivery of hydrophobic drugs. The main method of their preparation depends on solidification of the produced nanoemulsion. SLNs were reported to have enhanced retinal permeation in addition to prolongation of drug ocular retention [5].

Nanostructured lipid carriers (NLCs) were introduced as next-generation lipid nanocarriers to overcome the limitations of SLNs, such as low drug loading capacity due to its expulsion by crystallization of lipids. NLCs are composed of both solid and liquid lipids and thereby have asymmetric structure, which prevents drug expulsion and brings about comparatively slower drug release [5].

The aqueous dispersion of lipid nanoparticles is mainly applied topically for delivery of the entrapped medication to the anterior segment of the eye. The aim of the use of this nanocarrier is to prolong retention time at surface of the cornea by muco-adhesion as well as enhance corneal permeation.

For this purpose, cationic lipid nanoparticles were prepared by using cationic lipids [14, 15] that can interact with the negatively charged mucus. Additionally, coating lipid nanoparticles with bio-adhesive polymers such as hydroxypropyl methyl cellulose [16], hyaluronic acid [17], and chitosan [18–20] was also employed.

For example, Wang et al. [18] prepared chitosan-coated solid lipid nanoparticles loaded with methazolamide for glaucoma treatment. Their findings proved the enhanced lowering in intraocular pressure effect of the coated formulation compared with either the uncoated one or a commercial methazolamide eye drop.

Furthermore, the lipid nanocarrier could be incorporated in a thermo-sensitive gel aiming to increase corneal contact time [20].

Nanostructured lipid carriers as well have gained popularity in ocular drug delivery [21–25]. They were reported as an efficient drug delivery system for the posterior segment of the eye due to their lipid nature, high drug-loading capacity, and enhanced trans-corneal penetration [5]. For instance, palmitoylethanolamide-loaded nanostructured lipid carrier was prepared for treatment of diabetic retinopathy in rat model [25]. In-vivo evaluation of the developed system confirmed its ability to reach the retina upon topical administration as evidenced by the significant inhibition in the levels of retinal tumor necrosis factor-α compared with the free drug in diabetic rats [25].

5.4 Nanosuspensions

Nanosuspensions are a nanometric colloidal dispersions of hydrophobic drugs stabilized by polymers or surfactants. The ocular bioavailability of many hydrophobic drugs could be improved using nanosuspension technology via increasing their retention time [26]. Numerous corticosteroids such as prednisolone, dexamethasone [27], and hydrocortisone [27, 28] were formulated as nanosuspensions for their anti-inflammatory effect in the anterior eye segment. This resulted in elimination of the expected adverse effects associated with administration of large doses of theses corticosteroids such as production of glaucoma, cataract, and the most serious optic nerve degeneration [27]. Moreover, other drugs such as the cyclosporine [29] and antibacterial sparfloxacin [30] demonstrated a sustained drug release profile with better therapeutic efficacy when prepared as in nanosuspension form.

5.5 Vesicular delivery systems

5.5.1 Liposomes

They are spherical lipid vesicles composed mainly of phospholipids and cholesterol. A good biocompatibility, sustained release properties together with their ability to encapsulate both hydrophobic and hydrophilic drugs make liposomes ideal candidates for ocular drug delivery to both anterior and posterior segments of the eye [26]. Liposomes as an ocular delivery system were first introduced in 1981 for the delivery of the antiviral idoxuridine for treatment of keratitis [31]. Afterward, they were widely used to deliver various drugs to the eye.

For anterior eye disorders, Cyclosporine A-liposomes showed a significantly higher AUC $_{0–24\,h}$ in rabbits tears film compared with Restasis® (commercial cyclosporin A emulsion) with lower irritation potential [32]. Additionally, ciprofloxacin loaded liposomes exhibited a three-fold increase in ocular bioavailability in rabbits when compared with Ciprocin® eye drops [33]. Similarly, in-vivo evaluation of cationic liposomes containing ibuprofen versus ibuprofen eye drops revealed improved precorneal retention time and ocular bioavailability [34].

For posterior eye disorders, liposomes were extensively studied for effective drug delivery to the back of the eye. For instance, a novel liposomal formulation succeeded to enhance the bioavailability of flurbiprofen by 11.3 times compared with the free drug in the vitreous humor after intravitreal injection in rabbits [35]. In addition, the use of multivesicular liposomes to deliver the antibody Bevacizumab to the posterior eye chamber after intravitreal injection in rabbits was reported in treatment of choroidal neovascularization [36]. The elaborated system demonstrated an increase in intravitreal retention time as confirmed by in-vivo imaging of rat vitreous cavity, and hence the number of injection times was reduced [36]. Interestingly, the topical application of triamcinolone acetonide loaded chitosan-coated liposomes achieved better therapeutic outcomes in management of retinal edema instead of intravitreal injection of the drug [37, 38].

Despite the huge research conducted in the field of liposomal ocular drug delivery, their industrial production is limited owing to poor long-term stability, limited drug loading capacity, and difficulty during sterilization [6].

5.5.2 Niosomes

Niosomes were developed to overcome the limitations encountered by liposomes. Similar to liposomes, they are nontoxic vesicles and can encapsulate both hydrophilic and hydrophobic drugs, but they are chemically stable and do not require special techniques for handling. Niosomes are submicron-sized non-ionic surfactant vesicles that have potential applications in ocular drug delivery [39].

There are tremendous research articles reporting the use of niosomes in ocular therapy. Niosomes have been investigated for the ocular delivery of wide range of drugs such as anticholinergic drugs, anti-inflammatory drugs, anti-glaucoma drugs, and antibiotics [40].

To name a few, the antibacterial vancomycin was incorporated in niosomes integrated in pH-sensitive in-situ gel aiming to minimize drug-induced ocular irritation and prolong its effect [41]. The prepared formulation succeeded to eradicate infection with methicillin-resistant *Staphylococcus aureus* infection in rabbits as confirmed by the increase in the antibacterial effect by 180- and 2.5-fold compared with untreated animals and those treated with free drug solution, respectively [41].

For glaucoma management, latanoprost-loaded niosomes in thermo-sensitive Pluronic® F127 gel were developed [42]. The in-vivo evaluation of the prepared gel in rabbits confirmed its biocompatibility besides its longer duration of action (3 days) as compared with the commercial eye drops [42].

5.5.3 Discosomes

Discosomes are considered as modified niosomal formulations. They differ from niosomes by the addition of solulan C24 (non-ionic surfactant derived from lanolin). Interestingly, their large size (12–16 μm) prevents their drainage into the systemic circulation. Furthermore, their disc shape guarantees better fitting into the conjunctival sac [2]. Discosomes were reported to entrap larger quantity of timolol maleate compared with niosomes, thus increasing ocular bioavailability [43].

5.5.4 Spanlastics

They are elastic span containing vesicles that are composed of non-ionic surfactants (Span 40/60/80) and edge activators (sodium taurocholate, sodium deoxycholate, and Tween 80). The edge activators are responsible for providing flexibility to these vesicles. In addition, they were reported to be non-irritant and safe for ocular use. Furthermore, they are superior to niosomes in being highly deformable and thus can effectively deliver the entrapped drugs to the posterior eye segment. Therefore, the topical instillation of spanlastics can replace the intravitreal injections and hence increase patient compliance [44].

For instance, ketoconazole-loaded spanlastics demonstrated two times better corneal permeation compared with the niosomal formulation [45]. Fluorescently labeled spanlastics were detected in the virtuous humor of the rabbit's eye after 2 hours from topical instillation confirming their entry to the back of the eye. Similar observations were reported for the use spanlastics to deliver fluconazole, which showed enhanced permeability coefficient compared with either niosomes or Zocon ® eye drops [46].

6. New and advanced ocular drug delivery systems

6.1 Contact lenses

They are thin curved plastic lenses of disc shape that are placed on the cornea. Drug-releasing contact lenses are considered as drug reservoirs that permit continuous drug release near the tear fluid [47]. The first and most frequently used polymer for the manufacture of these lenses was poly hydroxy ethyl methacrylate cross-linked with ethylene glycol dimethyl acrylate. Recently, the use of silicone lenses was employed. Substantial research was conducted on the use of lenses as a drug carrier for ocular delivery. For example, they were investigated for many drugs such as ciprofloxacin [48], cyclosporine [49], dexamethasone [50], timolol [51], antifungal drugs [52], among others. Drug-eluting lenses were reported to increase drugs ocular bioavailability via prolongation of their duration of action and increase their corneal penetration [47].

Various methods of loading drugs on the contact lenses were reported. The simplest method is soaking the lenses with the drug solution. However, this method suffers from many limitations such as low drug loading capacity and rapid drug release within few hours failing to provide extended drug release [51]. In this context, Wei et al. [51] studied the effect of encapsulation of the antiglaucoma drug, timolol, into microemulsion before loading on contact lenses by soaking on the drug loading efficiency versus soaking the lenses with free drug solution. The use of microemulsion technology achieved a two-fold improvement in loading efficiency with sustained drug release pattern up to 48–96 h. In addition, it provided prolonged reduction in the intraocular pressure for 96 h in rabbit model for glaucoma. Additionally, they reported that the entrapment of timolol in microemulsion before loading on contact lenses did not alter either the swelling or the transmittance of the developed lenses [51]. Similar findings were reported for the ability of liposomes [53] or polymeric nanoparticles [54] to extend and control the release rate of the entrapped drugs from the contact lenses.

It is also worth mentioning that Johnson & Johnson company lunched Acuvue® Theravision™ (etafilcon A drug-eluting contact lens with ketotifen). This product is the world's first and only drug-eluting contact lenses indicated for prevention of ocular itching due to allergic conjunctivitis upon daily application. Additionally, this product is used for vision correction in patients having no red eyes [55].

6.2 Implants

Implants are a solid form of a drug that is intended to achieve controlled drug release over an extended period of time. The implants can be surgically inserted in the subconjunctival, epidural, or vitreous areas. They provide sustained and localized drug delivery with higher patient compliance compared with the topical drops [47].

Surodex ® (Oculex Pharmaceuticals, Inc., Sunnyvale, CA, USA) is a dexamethasone containing a biodegradable implant (1×5 mm) made of poly (lactic-co-glycolic acid). It is inserted in the anterior segment of the eye for the relief of inflammation after cataract surgeries. The drug is released at a constant rate for 7–10 days [47].

Lux Biosciences produced a silicone-based episcleral implant (LX201) for delivery of cyclosporine-A to the anterior chamber of the eye for 1 year. LX 201 is also being assessed in phase III clinical trials for prevention of corneal graft rejection [47].

Vitrasert® (Bausch & Laumb, Inc.) is the first intravitreal delivery system loaded with ganciclovir for treatment of cytomegalovirus retinitis. It is designed to release the drug over a period of 6–8 month [47].

Retisert® is another intravitreal implant (Bausch & Laumb, Inc.) that can release fluocinolone acetonide up to 3 years into the vitreous humor. It is approved for treatment of posterior uveitis [47].

Fluocinolone acetonide is also included in the Iluvien® intravitreal implant (Alimera Sciences, Inc.). It is indicated for treatment of diabetic macular edema.

Iluvien is being assessed in phase II clinical trials for its efficacy in dry and wet age-related macular degeneration as well as macular edema secondary to retinal vein occlusion compared with Lucentis® injection containing ranibizumab [47].

The Ozurdex® intravitreal dexamethasone implant is designed to release the drug for 3–6 months. It is approved for use in diabetic macular edema, posterior uveitis, and retinal vein occlusion [47].

Recently, a lot of sustained-release intraocular implants have been developed for glaucoma treatment. For example, Durysta™ (Allergan plc, Dublin, Ireland) is bimatoprost implant, which was approved by FDA in March 2020 for treatment of open-angle glaucoma and ocular hypertension. It can provide a sustained drug release up to 3–4 months [56]. Another example is the iDose® implant (Glaukos, California, USA) containing travoprost. It is a titanium implant of dimensions 1.8 mm x 0.5 m that is anchored within the trabecular meshwork. It achieves a zero-order drug release over a period of 6 months or longer. It showed promising results in phase II clinical trials versus topical solution of 0.5% timolol. Currently, the recruitment of patients for phase III clinical studies has started [56].

6.3 Microneedles

Microneedles (MNs) are a revolutionary delivery method that facilitates drug delivery to a variety of eye ailments with potential healthcare applications. MNs now allow localized, effective, less invasive, and targeted drug delivery in the eye. MNs were originally created as a painless, minimally invasive, and effective transdermal medication conveyance technique [57].

Microneedle applications on various ocular targets of the suprachoroid space of the rabbit eye [58, 59], the cornea of the mouse eye [60], and the sclera of a human cadaver eye [61] have been reported.

The use of MN in the eye may also have numerous advantages over invasive intra-ocular injections using long, typical hypodermic needles. MNs possess long enough dimensions to pass through the ocular obstacles of both the anterior and posterior sectors of the eye, allowing for targeted administration to the sclera, stroma, and suprachoroidal area [62].

MNs, as opposed to hypodermic needles, lower the risk of pain, tissue injury, and infection. Because little research has been done in this field, using MNs in ocular drug delivery is a relatively novel approach.

Applying MNs to biological membranes can establish microdimensional transport channels and improve drug penetration across biological membrane boundaries. They're produced from a variety of materials, such as silicon, stainless steel, glass, and polymers, and available in a variety of shapes, including solid and hollow design [63]. Many techniques such as micro molding, laser drilling, and lithography can be used to fabricate microneedles [63].

Using MNs, it's possible to deposit medicines or drug delivery systems into the sclera or the suprachoroidal region, which is the space between the sclera and the choroid (SCS). Micropuncturing the sclera layer may allow for more drugs or drug carriers to be deposited in the sclera, resulting in enhanced drug permeation into the deeper ocular tissues [64].

To inject particles of sizes 20–100 nm, a minimum pressure of 250 kPa and a minimum microneedle length of 800 μm should be maintained; on the other hand, a minimum pressure of 300 kPa and a needle length of 1000 μm are required for particles sizes between 500 and 1000 nm to penetrate the sclera [65].

Numerous research studies, according to Gupta and Yadava, have lately shown the use of MNs in ocular diseases such as glaucoma, age-related macular degeneration, uveitis, retinal vascular occlusion, retinitis pigmentosa, and others [66].

Patel et al. invented the hollow MN, which was injected into the SCS using a hollow glass microneedle [67]. SCS targeting allows for precise dosing and reduces medication exposure to non-targeted tissues. Patel et al. showed that clearance of molecules and particles injected into the SCS occurred at varying speeds depending on their size in a rabbit cadaver model [58].

Thakur et al. in 2014 utilized hollow MN devices of heights of 400, 500, and 600 μm made from hypodermic needles. These hollow MNs were used to inject a thermo-responsive poloxamer-based hydrogel containing sodium fluorescein as a model drug into the scleral tissue of a rabbit to form an in-situ implant within the micro-channels, resulting in a sustained release of fluorescein sodium over 24 hours in an in-vitro experiment. This type of implant production, which does not require surgery, would improve patient acceptability and could also deliver sustained medication levels, decreasing the need for frequent application of eye drops [68].

For targeted drug delivery, intrascleral hollow microneedles are being created. These microneedles can transport medications into the posterior portion of the eye via suprachoroidal, subconjunctival, and transcleral pathways. This delivery method can transfer nanoparticles, microparticles, and drugs solutions in a less intrusive way. However, to distribute microparticles, administration must be accompanied with spreading enzymes such as hyaluronidase and collagenase, which aid in the quick hydrolysis of the sclera's collagenous and extracellular matrix structure [69].

Datta et al. developed a fast-dissolving polyvinyl pyrrolidone MN ocular patch to deliver cyclosporin-A (CsA) to the cornea. CsA diffuses slowly into deeper ocular tissues and promote drug retention in the excised porcine cornea and resulted in effective ocular administration [70].

Dissolvable polyvinyl alcohol and polyvinyl pyrrolidone matrix were used to produce a dissolving microneedle ocular patch in the shape of a contact lens. These MNs, which include either amphotericin B loaded liposome or free amphotericin B, were found to be efficient in treating *Candida albicans* infection in both ex-vivo and rabbit models as well as improving corneal membrane epithelial and stromal differentiation [71].

In 2022, Shi et al. created a dissolving microneedle array patch based on poly(D,L-lactide) (PLA) and hyaluronic acid (HA) and containing fluconazole to develop a minimally invasive delivery system for treating fungal keratitis (FK). Interestingly, the rabbit model of FK reveals that the medicated topical MN patch has superior effect compared with the traditional eye drop formulation and is also equivalent to the clinical intrastromal injection technique [72].

For treatment of corneal neovascularization, a flexible double-layer microreservoir polymeric eye patch with a row of biodegradable detachable microneedles demonstrated to be more effective than topical eye drops. These biodegradable microneedles can penetrate through ocular barriers and self-implanted as a drug reservoir matrix for controlled drug release. Furthermore, rapid diclofenac release followed by extended monoclonal antibody release produces a synergistic effect in the treatment of corneal neovascularization [60].

In conclusion, MNs are thought to have the capacity to deliver other substances such as protein pharmaceuticals and DNA across the corneal epithelium with excellent effectiveness, which needs further exploration. MNs may serve as micro-drug reservoirs for targeted, regulated, and efficient ocular medication administration.

MNs are acceptable, harmless, and painless approach, resulting in a cost-effective treatment for a variety of ocular disorders.

6.4 Cell-based ocular therapy

Cell therapy is used to treat retinal degenerative illnesses by injecting cells into the subretina, usually with a microcatheter. Generally, in this method stem cells were injected into the retinal layers to stimulate cell regeneration. While animal studies imply that this approach is safe and nontoxic, the significant risk of consequences is an important concern [73]. Recently, Gandhi et al. have showed the safety and efficacy of degradable fibrin hydrogels for subretinal implantation to aid in the accurate implantation of retinal pigment epithelium monolayer. These promising hydrogels completely disintegrated after 8 weeks, making them the first fully biodegradable scaffold designed to treat macular degeneration disease [74].

6.5 Gene-based ocular delivery systems

The practice of transferring genetic material to remove, replace, repair, or introduce a gene to treat disorders is known as gene therapy [75]. Viral vectors, naked DNA, and nonviral vectors such as nanoparticles, microinjection, electroporation, sonoporation, and iontophoresis might all be used to deliver genes. Furthermore, cutting-edge approaches such as Genome Editing System, CRISPR-Cas Delivery, and siRNA treatment have been examined [76].

Retrovirus, adenovirus, and lentivirus are viral vectors that have shown excellent potential for transgene delivery to target cells in the eye because of the high transduction efficacy [75]. Kopone et al. reported that intraocular gene therapy for neovascularization has been found to be safe in clinical trials, with no serious side effects. Clinical trials, however, have not progressed beyond Phase II trials [75].

Although there are benefits to employing viral vectors, there are also numerous constraints. Preexisting immunity to viral vehicles (e.g., adenovirus) is a major concern, since it may result in low transduction rates and reduced expression of the therapeutic gene within cells. Furthermore, the residual viral proteins have the potential to trigger inflammation in their intended target [77].

Naked DNA can be used for gene therapy without a vector; however, its structural instability may limit adequate cell uptake [76]. Stechschulte et al. reported that naked DNA delivery to the cornea was safe, effective, titratable, and has the potential to alter the treatment of a wide variety of corneal and anterior segment diseases [78].

Nonviral vectors including metal [79], polymeric [80], lipid nanoparticle [81], and dendrimers [82] are also employed to deliver therapeutic genes to cells in the anterior and posterior portions of the eye. Nonviral vectors, in contrast to viral vectors, have been demonstrated to be more biologically safe, with reduced immunogenicity and pathogenicity. Nonviral vectors also have the advantage of being inexpensive and easy to produce. However, nonviral vehicles may have a lower transfection yield [83].

Physical methods are also applied to force DNA cellular entry, such as microinjection, electroporation, sonophoresis, and iontophoresis.

To facilitate plasmid gene transfer, electroporation uses high-intensity electric impulses to create pores within the cell membrane. To avoid corneal injury, edema, or inflammation, the ideal electrical field strength for this type of gene transfer is 200 V/cm. When compared with DNA injection alone, gene transfer in the cornea is 1000-fold higher [84].

On the other hand, sonoporation uses ultrasound waves to physically create transitory and limited pores inside cell membranes, allowing DNA to be transferred to the nucleus. Sonoporation can improve the amount of therapeutic gene expression by up to 15-fold when compared with naked DNA [85].

Concerning iontophoresis, it is a technique that uses low currents to create transitory and localized pores in the cell membrane, allowing ionized molecules to pass through. Iontophoresis has been shown to boost gene or drug transport across the cell membrane by 2.3 and 2.5 times in the cornea and 4.0 and 3.4 times in the conjunctiva, respectively; however, after the current was removed, the transfer recovered to baseline levels in rabbit cornea and conjunctiva [86].

Small interfering RNAs (siRNAs) are a type of non-coding, double-stranded RNA molecules with about 20–25 base pairs in length that influence mRNA gene expression. Several eye diseases have been treated with siRNAs, including retinal abnormalities, glaucoma, wound healing, and neovascularization [87]. The majority of these research used animal models, while some were evaluated in human disorders and other siRNAs still under clinical trials [88].

CRISPR-Cas9 genome editing is becoming a hot topic in gene therapy [76]. The effectiveness demonstrated in delivering this gene-editing system to the posterior eye [89] via viral and nonviral approaches provides a starting guide for additional research concerning anterior segment diseases.

In conclusion, the future development of efficient gene treatments will rely on a better knowledge of the mutations and mechanisms that cause visual abnormalities, as well as the development of more efficient clinical vectors.

6.6 Drug-device combinations used for ocular diseases

Several drug devices and combinations have been designed to improve drug delivery to the eye, but only a few have reached the market. They boost medication retention and penetration while allowing for long-term drug release. They also have a lower level of toxicity and better patient compliance. Genes, drugs, and cell-based pharmaceuticals, as well as their combinations with medical devices, all fall within the category of advanced therapeutics medicinal products (ATMPs).

In 2017, Rupenthal reported that devices, namely collagen shield and contact lenses that gradually dissolve into a gel are effective for dry eye management and enhance wound healing after corneal surgery. They're also employed as antibiotic and anti-inflammatory medicine reservoirs before and after surgery [90].

Yellepeddi et al. described a device known as punctal plugs (PPs) that prevents tears from draining via the canaliculi, which connects the eye to the nose. PPs are recommended in some cases of laser in situ keratomileusis and contact lens intolerance due to their capacity to preserve tears. The insertion of PPs has also been shown to increase tear film stability, tear osmolarity, and functional visual sharpness in dry eye patients. Silicone has been used to create PP designs. Another example produced by (Medenium, CA, USA) and commercialized as SmartPLUG™ was designed to improve PP retention in the puncta. SmartPLUG™ comprises a biocompatible hydrophobic thermosensitive copolymer [91].

In another study, PPs loaded with the antibiotic moxifloxacin (Ocular Therapeutix, MA, USA) were produced for prolonged drug administration in the treatment of bacterial conjunctivitis [92].

Eibl-Lindner and coworkers created erufosine-loaded intraocular lenses (IOLs) for prophylaxis against posterior capsule opacification. They stated that the designed IOP could have a therapeutic potential. They also reported that heparin-coated IOLs could be useful for reducing intraocular inflammation after cataract surgery [93].

Some of the devices mentioned in the literature are studied in clinical trials. For example, a live-cell delivery system that allows ciliary neurotrophic factor to be released from genetically engineered retinal pigment epithelium (RPE) cells. Implants utilizing this technique, designated as "Encapsulated Cell TechnologyR" (ECT) by the production company, have been shown to deliver protein drugs efficiently. ECT is made up of live cells loaded in an implanted matrix that acts as a medical device, allowing proteins generated by the cells to enter the body's fluids.

Finally, we can assert that manufacturing these devices under a pharmaceutical quality assurance system is a crucial step toward a faster production and efficient clinical application. This necessitates the formation of diverse research teams as well as the creation of infrastructure that adheres to GMP standards and meets the regulatory requirements of pharmaceutical quality systems.

7. Conclusions

The development of innovative, noninvasive, safe, and patient-compliant drug delivery techniques is the focus of intense ocular research.

Numerous drug delivery carrier systems utilizing nanotechnology, cell-based systems, microneedles, contact lenses, implants, and different devices are being developed. Ocular gene therapy has recently emerged as a promising method for treating, curing, or preventing diseases by altering the gene expression in the eyes. However, the creation of future effective treatments using gene delivery will depend on a deeper comprehension of the mutations that lead to visual impairments.

Assessment of in-vivo effect utilizing ocular models of cell lines may help to further generate accurate data at the preclinical and clinical phases since many ocular drug delivery studies are only confined to in-vitro performances.

In spite of numerous research articles published in this field, there is still a large gap in the study on ocular therapeutic systems. The absence of valid and reliable ex-vivo models that can accurately simulate the physiology of the ocular tissues is the main essential obstacle to establishing highly optimized ocular drug delivery systems.

Finally, we might anticipate that within the next 10 years, the market would have a significant increase in the development of novel drug delivery technologies due to the pace at which ocular research and efforts are being done.

DOI: http://dx.doi.org/10.5772/intechopen.106335

Author details

Amal H. El-Kamel* and Asmaa A. Ashour
Faculty of Pharmacy, Department of Pharmaceutics, Alexandria University, Alexandria, Egypt

*Address all correspondence to: amalelkamel@alexu.edu.eg

References

[1] Wang R, Gao Y, Liu A, Zhai G. A review of nanocarrier-mediated drug delivery systems for posterior segment eye disease: Challenges analysis and recent advances. Journal of Drug Targeting. 2021;**7**:687-702. DOI: 10.1080/1061186X.2021.1878366

[2] Suri R, Beg S, Kohli K. Target strategies for drug delivery bypassing ocular barriers. Journal of Drug Delivery Science and Technology. 2020;**55**:101389. DOI: 10.1016/j.jddst.2019.101389

[3] Agrahari V, Mandal A, Agrahari V, Trinh HM, Joseph M, Ray A, et al. A comprehensive insight on ocular pharmacokinetics. Drug Delivery and Translational Research. 2016;**6**:735-754. DOI: 10.1007/s13346-016-0339-2

[4] Fayyaz A, Vellonen KS, Ranta VP, Toropainen E, Reinisalo M, Valtari A, et al. Ocular pharmacokinetics of atenolol, timolol and betaxolol cocktail: Tissue exposures in the rabbit eye. European Journal of Pharmaceutics and Biopharmaceutics. 2021;**166**:155-162. DOI: 10.1016/j.ejpb.2021.06.003

[5] Gorantla S, Rapalli VK, Waghule T, Singh PP, Dubey SK, Saha RN, et al. Nanocarriers for ocular drug delivery: Current status and translational opportunity. RSC Advances. 2020;**10**(46):27835-27855. DOI: 10.1039/d0ra04971a

[6] Zhang J, Jiao J, Niu M, Gao X, Zhang G, Yu H, et al. Ten years of knowledge of nano-carrier based drug delivery systems in ophthalmology: Current evidence, challenges, and future prospective. International Journal of Nanomedicine. 2021;**16**:6497-6530. DOI: 10.2147/IJN.S329831

[7] Gote V, Ansong M, Pal D. Prodrugs and nanomicelles to overcome ocular barriers for drug penetration. Expert Opinion on Drug Metabolism & Toxicology. 2020;**16**(10):885-906. DOI: 10.1080/17425255.2020.1803278

[8] Cholkar K, Gilger BC, Mitra AK. Topical, aqueous, clear cyclosporine formulation design for anterior and posterior ocular delivery. Translational Vision Science & Technology. 2015;**4**(3):1. DOI: 10.1167/tvst.4.3.1

[9] Safwat MA, Mansour HF, Hussein AK, Abdelwahab S, Soliman GM. Polymeric micelles for the ocular delivery of triamcinolone acetonide: Preparation and in vivo evaluation in a rabbit ocular inflammatory model. Drug Delivery. 2020;**27**(1):1115-1124. DOI: 10.1080/10717544.2020.1797241

[10] Xu X, Sun L, Zhou L, Cheng Y, Cao F. Functional chitosan oligosaccharide nanomicelles for topical ocular drug delivery of dexamethasone. Carbohydrate Polymers. 2020;**227**:115356. DOI: 10.1016/j.carbpol.2019.115356

[11] Omerović N, Vranić E. Application of nanoparticles in ocular drug delivery systems. Health Technology. 2020;**10**:61-78. DOI: 10.1007/s12553-019-00381-w

[12] Radwan SE, El-Moslemany RM, Mehanna RA, Thabet EH, Abdelfattah EA, El-Kamel A. Chitosan-coated bovine serum albumin nanoparticles for topical tetrandrine delivery in glaucoma: In vitro and in vivo assessment. Drug Delivery. 2022;**29**(1):1150-1163. DOI: 10.1080/10717544.2022.2058648

[13] Radwan SE, El-Kamel A, Zaki EI, Burgalassi S, Zucchetti E,

El-Moslemany RM. Hyaluronic-coated albumin nanoparticles for the non-invasive delivery of apatinib in diabetic retinopathy. International Journal of Nanomedicine. 2021;**16**:4481-4494. DOI: 10.2147/IJN.S316564

[14] Başaran E, Demirel M, Sirmagül B, Yazan Y. Cyclosporine-A incorporated cationic solid lipid nanoparticles for ocular delivery. Journal of Microencapsulation. 2010;**27**(1):37-47. DOI: 10.3109/02652040902846883

[15] Leonardi A, Bucolo C, Drago F, Salomone SR. P. Cationic solid lipid nanoparticles enhance ocular hypotensive effect of melatonin in rabbit. International Journal of Pharmaceutics. 2015;**478**(1):180-186. DOI: 10.1016/j.ijpharm.2014.11.032

[16] Kiss EL, Berkó S, Gácsi A, Kovács A, Katona G, Soós J, et al. Development and characterization of potential ocular mucoadhesive nano lipid carriers using full factorial design. Pharmaceutics. 2020;**12**(7):682. DOI: 10.3390/pharmaceutics12070682

[17] Apaolaza PS, Delgado D, del Pozo-Rodríguez A, Gascón AR. and Solinís MÁ.A novel gene therapy vector based on hyaluronic acid and solid lipid nanoparticles for ocular diseases. International Journal of Pharmaceutics. 2014;**465**(1-2):413-426. DOI: 10.1016/j.ijpharm.2014.02.038

[18] Wang F, Chen L, Zhang D, Jiang S, Shi K, Huang Y, et al. Methazolamide-loaded solid lipid nanoparticles modified with low-molecular weight chitosan for the treatment of glaucoma: In-vitro and in-vivo study. Journal of Drug Targeting. 2014;**22**(9):849-858. DOI: 10.3109/1061186X.2014.939983

[19] Eid HM, Elkomy MH, El Menshawe SF, Salem HF. Development, optimization, and in vitro/in vivo characterization of enhanced lipid nanoparticles for ocular delivery of ofloxacin: The influence of pegylation and chitosan coating. AAPS PharmSciTech. 2019;**20**(5):183. DOI: 10.1208/s12249-019-1371-6

[20] Eldesouky LM, El-Moslemany RM, Ramadan AA, Morsi MH, Khalafallah NM. Cyclosporine lipid nanocapsules as thermoresponsive gel for dry eye management: Promising corneal mucoadhesion, biodistribution and preclinical efficacy in rabbits. Pharmaceutics. 2021;**13**(3):360. DOI: 10.3390/pharmaceutics13030360

[21] Lakhani P, Patil A, Taskar P, Ashour E, Majumdar S. Curcumin-loaded nanostructured lipid carriers for ocular drug delivery: Design optimization and characterization. Journal of Drug Delivery Science and Technology. 2018;**47**:159-166. DOI: 10.1016/j.jddst.2018.07.010

[22] Patil A, Lakhani P, Taskar P, Wu KW, Sweeney C, Avula B, et al. Formulation development, optimization, and in vitro-in vivo characterization of natamycin-loaded pegylated nano-lipid carriers for ocular applications. Journal of Pharmaceutical Sciences. 2018;**107**(8):2160-2171. DOI: 10.1016/j.xphs.2018.04.014

[23] Selvaraj K, Kuppusamy G, Krishnamurthy J, Mahalingam R, Singh SK, Gulati M. Repositioning of itraconazole for the management of ocular neovascularization through surface-modified nanostructured lipid carriers. Assay and Drug Development Technologies. 2019;**17**(4):178-190. DOI: 10.1089/adt.2018.898

[24] Rathod VR, Shah DA, Dave RH. Systematic implementation of quality-by-design (QbD) to develop NSAID-loaded

nanostructured lipid carriers for ocular application: Preformulation screening studies and statistical hybrid-design for optimization of variables. Drug Development and Industrial Pharmacy. 2020;**46**(3):443-455. DOI: 10.1080/03639045.2020.1724135

[25] Puglia C, Santonocito D, OstacoloC,MariaSommellaE,CampigliaP, Carbone C, et al. Ocular formulation based on palmitoylethanolamide-loaded nanostructured lipid carriers: Technological and pharmacological profile. Nanomaterials (Basel). 2020;**10**(2):287. DOI: 10.3390/nano10020287

[26] Kamaleddin MA. Nano-ophthalmology: Applications and considerations. Nanomedicine. 2017;**13**(4):1459-1472. DOI: 10.1016/j.nano.2017.02.007

[27] Kassem MA, Abdel Rahman AA, Ghorab MM, Ahmed MB, Khalil RM. Nanosuspension as an ophthalmic delivery system for certain glucocorticoid drugs. International Journal of Pharmaceutics. 2007;**340**(1-2):126-133. DOI: 10.1016/j.ijpharm.2007.03.011

[28] Ali HS, York P, Ali AM, Blagden N. Hydrocortisone nanosuspensions for ophthalmic delivery: A comparative study between microfluidic nanoprecipitation and wet milling. Journal of Controlled Release. 2011;**149**(2):175-181. DOI: 10.1016/j.jconrel.2010.10.007

[29] Yan R, Xu L, Wang Q, Wu Z, Zhang H, Gan L. Cyclosporine a nanosuspensions for ophthalmic delivery: A comparative study between cationic nanoparticles and drug-core mucus penetrating nanoparticles. Molecular Pharmaceutics. 2021;**18**(12):4290-4298. DOI: 10.1021/acs.molpharmaceut.1c00370

[30] Ambhore NP, Dandagi PM, Gadad AP. Formulation and comparative evaluation of HPMC and water soluble chitosan-based sparfloxacin nanosuspension for ophthalmic delivery. Drug Delivery and Translational Research. 2016;**6**(1):48-56. DOI: 10.1007/s13346-015-0262-y

[31] Smolin G, Okumoto M, Feiler S, Condon D. Idoxuridine-liposome therapy for herpes simplex keratitis. American Journal of Ophthalmology. 1981;**91**(2):220-225. DOI: 10.1016/0002-9394(81)90177-x

[32] Karn PR, Kim HD, Kang H, Sun BK, Jin SE, Hwang SJ. Supercritical fluid-mediated liposomes containing cyclosporin A for the treatment of dry eye syndrome in a rabbit model: Comparative study with the conventional cyclosporin A emulsion. International Journal of Nanomedicine. 2014;**9**:3791-3800. DOI: 10.2147/IJN.S65601

[33] Taha EI, El-Anazi MH, El-Bagory IM, Bayomi MA. Design of liposomal colloidal systems for ocular delivery of ciprofloxacin. Saudi Pharmaceutical Journal. 2014;**22**(3):231-239. DOI: 10.1016/j.jsps.2013.07.003

[34] Gai X, Cheng L, Li T, Liu D, Wang Y, Wang T, et al. In vitro and in vivo studies on a novel bioadhesive colloidal system: Cationic liposomes of ibuprofen. AAPS PharmSciTech. 2018;**19**(2):700-709. DOI: 10.1208/s12249-017-0872-4

[35] Blazaki S, Pachis K, Tzatzarakis M, Tsilimbaris M, Antimisiaris SG. Novel Liposome Aggregate Platform (LAP) system for sustained retention of drugs in the posterior ocular segment following intravitreal injection. International Journal of Pharmaceutics. 2020;**576**:118987. DOI: 10.1016/j.ijpharm.2019.118987

[36] Mu H, Wang Y, Chu Y, Jiang Y, Hua H, Chu L, et al. Multivesicular liposomes for sustained release of bevacizumab in treating laser-induced choroidal neovascularization. Drug Delivery. 2018;**25**(1):1372-1383. DOI: 10.1080/10717544.2018.1474967

[37] Cheng T, Li J, Cheng Y, Zhang X, Qu Y. Triamcinolone acetonide-chitosan coated liposomes efficiently treated retinal edema as eye drops. Experimental Eye Research. 2019;**188**:107805. DOI: 10.1016/j.exer.2019.107805

[38] Li J, Cheng T, Tian Q, Cheng Y, Zhao L, Zhang X, et al. A more efficient ocular delivery system of triamcinolone acetonide as eye drop to the posterior segment of the eye. Drug Delivery. 2019;**26**(1):188-198. DOI: 10.1080/10717544.2019.1571122

[39] Durak S, Esmaeili Rad M, Alp Yetisgin A, Eda Sutova H, Kutlu O, Cetinel S, et al. Niosomal drug delivery systems for ocular disease-recent advances and future prospects. Nanomaterials (Basel). 2020;**10**(6):1191. DOI: 10.3390/nano10061191

[40] Verma A, Tiwari A, Saraf S, Panda PK, Jain A, Jain SK. Emerging potential of niosomes in ocular delivery. Expert Opinion on Drug Delivery. 2021;**18**(1):55-71. DOI: 10.1080/17425247.2020.1822322

[41] Allam A, El-Mokhtar MA, Elsabahy M. Vancomycin-loaded niosomes integrated within pH-sensitive in-situ forming gel for treatment of ocular infections while minimizing drug irritation. The Journal of Pharmacy and Pharmacology. 2019;**71**(8):1209-1221. DOI: 10.1111/jphp.13106

[42] Fathalla D, Fouad EA, Soliman GM. Latanoprost niosomes as a sustained release ocular delivery system for the management of glaucoma. Drug Development and Industrial Pharmacy. 2020;**46**(5):806-813. DOI: 10.1080/03639045.2020.1755305

[43] Vyas SP, Mysore N, Jaitely V, Venkatesan N. Discoidal niosome based controlled ocular delivery of timolol maleate. Die Pharmazie. 1998;**53**(7):466-469

[44] Chablani L and Kumar V. Nanovesicular carrier systems for ophthalmic drug delivery. In: Pathak Y, Sutariya V, Hiran A, editors. Nano-Biomaterials For Ophthalmic Drug Delivery. Springer, Cham; 2016. p. 231-242. DOI: 10.1007/978-3-319-29346-2_11. ch 11.

[45] Kakkar S, Kaur IP. Spanlastics-a novel nanovesicular carrier system for ocular delivery. International Journal of Pharmaceutics. 2011;**413**(1-2):202-210. DOI: 10.1016/j.ijpharm.2011.04.027

[46] Kaur IP, Rana C, Singh M, Bhushan S, Singh H, Kakkar S. Development and evaluation of novel surfactant-based elastic vesicular system for ocular delivery of fluconazole. Journal of Ocular Pharmacology and Therapeutics. 2012;**28**(5):484-496. DOI: 10.1089/jop.2011.0176

[47] Gote V, Sikder S, Sicotte J, Pal D. Ocular drug delivery: Present innovations and future challenges. The Journal of Pharmacology and Experimental Therapeutics. 2019;**370**(3):602-624. DOI: 10.1124/jpet.119.256933

[48] Hui A, Willcox M, Jones L. In vitro and in vivo evaluation of novel ciprofloxacin-releasing silicone hydrogel contact lenses. Investigative Ophthalmology & Visual Science. 2014;**55**(8):4896-4904. DOI: 10.1167/iovs.14-14855

[49] Choi JH, Li Y, Jin R, Shrestha T, Choi JS, Lee WJ, et al. The efficiency of cyclosporine a-eluting contact lenses for the treatment of dry eye. Current Eye Research. 2019;**44**(5):486-496. DOI: 10.1080/02713683.2018.1563702

[50] Bengani LC, Kobashi H, Ross AE, Zhai H, Salvador-Culla B, Tulsan R, et al. Steroid-eluting contact lenses for corneal and intraocular inflammation. Acta Biomaterialia. 2020;**116**:149-161. DOI: 10.1016/j.actbio.2020.08.013

[51] Wei N, Dang H, Huang C, Sheng Y. Timolol loaded microemulsion laden silicone contact lens to manage glaucoma: In vitro and in vivo studies.J Dispers. Science and Technology. 2021;**42**(5):742-750. DOI: 10.1080/01932691.2019.1710183

[52] Phan CM, Bajgrowicz M, McCanna DJ, Subbaraman LN, Jones L. Effects of antifungal soaked silicone hydrogel contact lenses on candida albicans in an agar eye model. Eye & Contact Lens. 2016;**42**(5):313-317. DOI: 10.1097/ICL.0000000000000209

[53] Danion A, Arsenault I, Vermette P. Antibacterial activity of contact lenses bearing surface-immobilized layers of intact liposomes loaded with levofloxacin. Journal of Pharmaceutical Sciences. 2007;**96**(9):2350-2363. DOI: 10.1002/jps.20871

[54] Nasr FH, Khoee S, Dehghan MM, Chaleshtori SS, Shafiee A. Preparation and evaluation of contact lenses embedded with polycaprolactone-based nanoparticles for ocular drug delivery. Biomacromolecules. 2016;**17**(2):485-495. DOI: 10.1021/acs.biomac.5b01387

[55] Yang Y, Lockwood A. Topical ocular drug delivery systems: Innovations for an unmet need. Experimental Eye Research. 2022;**218**:109006. DOI: 10.1016/j.exer.2022.109006

[56] Miller PE, Eaton JS. Medical anti-glaucoma therapy: Beyond the drop. Veterinary Ophthalmology. 2021;**24**(Suppl. 1):2-15. DOI: 10.1111/vop.12843

[57] Waghule T, Singhvi G, Dubey SK, Pandey MM, Gupta G, Singh M, et al. Microneedles: A smart approach and increasing potential for transdermal drug delivery system. Biomedicine & Pharmacotherapy. 2019;**109**:1249-1258. DOI: 10.1016/j.biopha.2018.10.078

[58] Patel SR, Berezovsky DE, McCarey BE, Zarnitsyn V, Edelhauser HF, Prausnitz MR. Targeted administration into the suprachoroidal space using a microneedle for drug delivery to the posterior segment of the eye. Investigative Ophthalmology & Visual Science. 2012;**53**(8):4433-4441. DOI: 10.1167/iovs.12-9872

[59] Chiang B, Venugopal N, Edelhauser HF, Prausnitz MR. Distribution of particles, small molecules and polymeric formulation excipients in the suprachoroidal space after microneedle injection. Experimental Eye Research. 2016;**153**:101-109. DOI: 10.1016/j.exer.2016.10.011

[60] Than A, Liu C, Chang H, Duong PK, Cheung CMG, Xu C, et al. Self-implantable double-layered micro-drug-reservoirs for efficient and controlled ocular drug delivery. Nature Communications. 2018;**9**(1):4433. DOI: 10.1038/s41467-018-06981-w

[61] Jiang J, Moore JS, Edelhauser HF, Prausnitz MR. Intrascleral drug delivery to the eye using hollow microneedles. Pharmaceutical Research. 2009;**26**(2):395-403. DOI: 10.1007/s11095-008-9756-3

[62] Thakur Singh RR, Tekko I, McAvoy K, McMillan H, Jones D,

Donnelly RF. Minimally invasive microneedles for ocular drug delivery. Expert Opinion on Drug Delivery. 2017;**14**(4):525-537. DOI: 10.1080/17425247.2016.1218460

[63] Wang R, Jiang G, Aharodnikau UE, Yunusov K, Sun Y, Liu T, et al. Recent advances in polymer microneedles for drug transdermal delivery: Design strategies and applications. Macromolecular Rapid Communications. 2022;**43**(8):e2200037. DOI: 10.1002/marc.202200037

[64] Donnelly RF, Raj Singh TR, Woolfson AD. Microneedle-based drug delivery systems: Microfabrication, drug delivery, and safety. Drug Delivery. 2010;**17**(4):187-207. DOI: 10.3109/10717541003667798

[65] Bennett L. Other. Advances in ocular drug delivery, in ocular drug delivery: Advances, challenges and applications, R.T. Addo, Editor. 2016, Springer International Publishing: Cham. p. 165-185. DOI: 10.1007/978-3-319-47691-9_10. Ch10.

[66] Gupta P, Yadav KS. Applications of microneedles in delivering drugs for various ocular diseases. Life Sciences. 2019;**237**:116907. DOI: 10.1016/j.lfs.2019.116907

[67] Patel SR, Lin AS, Edelhauser HF, Prausnitz MR. Suprachoroidal drug delivery to the back of the eye using hollow microneedles. Pharmaceutical Research. 2011;**28**(1):166-176. DOI: 10.1007/s11095-010-0271-y

[68] Thakur RR, Fallows SJ, McMillan HL, Donnelly RF, Jones DS. Microneedle-mediated intrascleral delivery of in situ forming thermoresponsive implants for sustained ocular drug delivery. The Journal of Pharmacy and Pharmacology. 2014;**66**(4):584-595. DOI: 10.1111/jphp.12152

[69] Balguri SP, Adelli GR, Majumdar S. Topical ophthalmic lipid nanoparticle formulations (SLN, NLC) of indomethacin for delivery to the posterior segment ocular tissues. European Journal of Pharmaceutics and Biopharmaceutics. 2016;**109**:224-235. DOI: 10.1016/j.ejpb.2016.10.015

[70] Datta D, Roy G, Garg P, Venuganti VV. Ocular delivery of cyclosporine A using dissolvable microneedle contact lens. Journal of Drug Delivery Science and Technology. 2022;**1**(70):103211. DOI: 10.1016/j.jddst.2022.103211

[71] Roy G, Galigama RD, Thorat VS, Mallela LS, Roy S, Garg P, et al. Amphotericin B containing microneedle ocular patch for effective treatment of fungal keratitis. International Journal of Pharmaceutics. 2019;**572**:118808. DOI: 10.1016/j.ijpharm.2019.118808

[72] Shi H, Zhou J, Wang Y, Zhu Y, Lin D, Lei L, et al. A rapid corneal healing microneedle for efficient ocular drug delivery. Small. 2022;**18**(4):e2104657. DOI: 10.1002/smll.202104657

[73] Kang-Mieler JJ, Rudeen KM, Liu W, Mieler WF. Advances in ocular drug delivery systems. Eye (London, England). 2020;**34**(8):1371-1379. DOI: 10.1038/s41433-020-0809-0

[74] Gandhi JK, Mano F, Iezzi R Jr, LoBue SA, Holman BH, Fautsch MP, et al. Fibrin hydrogels are safe, degradable scaffolds for sub-retinal implantation. PLoS One. 2020;**15**(1):e0227641. DOI: 10.1371/journal.pone.022764

[75] Koponen S, Kokki E, Kinnunen K, Ylä-Herttuala S. Viral-vector-delivered anti-angiogenic therapies to the eye. Pharmaceutics. 2021;**13**(2):219. DOI: 10.3390/pharmaceutics13020219

[76] Amador C, Shah R, Ghiam S, Kramerov AA, Ljubimov AV. Gene therapy in the anterior eye segment. Current Gene Therapy. 2022;**22**(2):104-131. DOI: 10.2174/1566523221666210423084233

[77] Shirley JL, de Jong YP, Terhorst C, Herzog RW. Immune responses to viral gene therapy vectors. Molecular Therapy. 2020;**28**(3):709-722. DOI: 10.1016/j.ymthe.2020.01.001

[78] Stechschulte SU, Joussen AM, von Recum HA, Poulaki V, Moromizato Y, Yuan J, et al. Rapid ocular angiogenic control via naked DNA delivery to cornea. Investigative Ophthalmology & Visual Science. 2001;**42**(9):1975-1979

[79] Masse F, Desjardins P, Ouellette M, Couture C, Omar MM, Pernet V, et al. Synthesis of ultrastable gold nanoparticles as a new drug delivery system. Molecules. 2019;**24**(16):2929. DOI: 10.3390/molecules24162929

[80] Tong YC, Chang SF, Kao WW, Liu CY, Liaw J. Polymeric micelle gene delivery of bcl-xL via eye drop reduced corneal apoptosis following epithelial debridement. Journal of Controlled Release. 2010;**147**(1):76-83. DOI: 10.1016/j.jconrel.2010.06.006

[81] Torrecilla J, Gómez-Aguado I, Vicente-Pascual M, Del Pozo-Rodríguez A. Solinís MÁ, and Rodríguez-Gascón A.MMP-9 Downregulation with Lipid Nanoparticles for Inhibiting Corneal Neovascularization by Gene Silencing. Nanomaterials (Basel). 2019;**9**(4):631. DOI: 10.3390/nano9040631

[82] Kalomiraki M, Thermos K, Chaniotakis NA. Dendrimers as tunable vectors of drug delivery systems and biomedical and ocular applications. International Journal of Nanomedicine. 2015;**11**:1-12. DOI: 10.2147/IJN.S93069

[83] Bordet T, Behar-Cohen F. Ocular gene therapies in clinical practice: viral vectors and nonviral alternatives. Drug Discovery Today. 2019;**24**(8):1685-1693. DOI: 10.1016/j.drudis.2019.05.038

[84] Blair-Parks K, Weston BC, Dean DA. High-level gene transfer to the cornea using electroporation. The Journal of Gene Medicine. 2002;**4**(1):92-100. DOI: 10.1002/jgm.231

[85] Wells DJ. Gene therapy progress and prospects: Electroporation and other physical methods. Gene Therapy. 2004;**11**(18):1363-1369. DOI: 10.1038/sj.gt.3302337

[86] Sekijima H, Ehara J, Hanabata Y, Suzuki T, Kimura S, Lee VH, et al. Characterization of ocular iontophoretic drug transport of ionic and non-ionic compounds in isolated rabbit cornea and conjunctiva. Biological & Pharmaceutical Bulletin. 2016;**39**(6):959-968. DOI: 10.1248/bpb.b15-00932

[87] Supe S, Upadhya A, Singh K. Role of small interfering RNA (siRNA) in targeting ocular neovascularization: A review. Experimental Eye Research. 2021;**202**:108329. DOI: 10.1016/j.exer.2020.108329

[88] Guzman-Aranguez A, Loma P, Pintor J. Small-interfering RNAs (siRNAs) as a promising tool for ocular therapy. British Journal of Pharmacology. 2013;**170**(4):730-747. DOI: 10.1111/bph.12330

[89] Lohia A, Sahel DK, Salman M, Singh V, Mariappan I, Mittal A, et al. Delivery strategies for CRISPR/Cas genome editing tool for retinal dystrophies: Challenges and opportunities.Asian. Journal of Pharmaceutical Sciences. 2022;**17**(2): 153-176. DOI: 10.1016/j.ajps.2022.02.001

[90] Rupenthal ID. Drug-device combination approaches for delivery to the eye. Current Opinion in Pharmacology. 2017;**36**:44-51. DOI: 10.1016/j.coph.2017.08.003

[91] Yellepeddi VK, Sheshala R, McMillan H, Gujral C, Jones D, Singh TRR. Punctal plug: A medical device to treat dry eye syndrome and for sustained drug delivery to the eye. Drug Discovery Today. 2015;**20**(7):884-889. DOI: 10.1016/j.drudis.2015.01.013

[92] Chee SP. Moxifloxacin punctum plug for sustained drug delivery. Journal of Ocular Pharmacology and Therapeutics. 2012;**28**(4):340-349. DOI: 10.1089/jop.2011.0162

[93] Eibl-Lindner KH, Wertheimer C, Die AK. Intraokularlinse als Arzneimittelträger: Stand der forschung und Ausblick [Intraocular Lens as a Drug Delivery Device: State of the Art and Future Perspective]. Klinische Monatsblätter für Augenheilkunde. 2016;**233**(2):172-178. German. DOI: 10.1055/s-0041-109512

Chapter 4

Recent Pharmaceutical Developments in the Treatment of Cancer Using Nanosponges

Kapil Gore, Sankha Bhattacharya and Bhupendra Prajapati

Abstract

Nanosponges are a class of nanoparticles characterized by their sponge-like surface that ensures high loading capacity. Cancer causes high mortality and requires precise treatment without harming the body. Hence, nanoparticles are required to target medications to tumor. Nanosponges may be synthesized from various polymers and metals, giving them distinct properties. The majority of polymer synthesis entails crosslinking, while metal synthesis entails the isolation of metal nanoparticles accompanied by their assembly into sponges. Nanosponges must be functionalized to precisely attack tumors. There are several patents on nanosponges synthesis and their use. Future trends in the usage of nanosponges include simultaneous distribution of several molecules and expanding the spectrum of use from medicinal delivery to substance encapsulation for a multitude of applications. As their usage in the pharmaceutical industry grows, more emphasis should be put on toxicity-related aspects induced by the near association of cell membrane and nanosponge resulting in intracellular dissolution or reactive oxygen species (ROS) generation, which in turn damages various cellular components. Many techniques have been created to reduce toxicity, including functionalization with various materials such as antioxidants, polymers and altering nanosponges composition. As the application of nanosponges increases in many industries, the phenomenon related to toxicity must be further explored through research.

Keywords: nanosponges, nanoparticles, silver nanosponges, cyclodextrin nanosponges, cancer therapy, β-hydroxypropyl beta-cyclodextrin

1. Introduction

Cancer is a collection of diseases triggered due to uncontrolled cell division [1]. Cancer cells are able to migrate from their original site to any other site through the vasculature is what that makes them harmful [2]. Cancer occupies the second position in list of deaths worldwide by causing 9.6 million deaths in 2018. Cancer causes a tremendous economic burden on the patient and ultimately on the nation [3]. Traditional treatments for cancer include surgery, chemotherapy and radiation therapy [4]. The traditional therapies are now more advanced as the time has progressed. Yet, they have many drawbacks which make them ineffective for destruction of tumor [5]. Surgical treatments suffer from disadvantages such as early diagnosis, presence of micro metastases, disruptions of tumors and side effects of anesthesia [6]. Radiotherapy involves treatment with ionizing radiations with a drawback of non-discriminate action against healthy cells at the sites where cells have a rapid growth rate such as hair follicles. It causes side effects like hair loss, anemia, sores in mouth and throat, neuropathy, skin dryness, and change in skin color [7]. To prevent these side effects, nanoparticles are used that can penetrate inside the tumor due to their nanosize. It reduces not only the amount of drug used but also the associated side effects due to action at places where it is not needed [8]. Many nano-formulations such as nanosponges and nanoparticles have been invented for their delivery to cancer [9]. In this chapter, we have discussed about nanosponges, their classification, advantages, disadvantages, and how they are better than other nanocarriers. We have also enlisted the barriers affecting delivery to cancer and how nanosponges can be used to overcome them along with some applications of nanosponges along with functionalization of nanosponges to ease delivery to cancer. We have also discussed about toxicity of nanosponges and the probable mechanisms to reduce that toxicity.

2. Nanoparticles in treatment of cancer

Nanoparticles are nanosized particles containing polymers or lipids which contain drugs adsorbed or encapsulated in them [10]. One advantage of nanotechnology in cancer treatment is modifications of delivery system to achieve targeting [11]. Nanoparticle-mediated delivery of any cytotoxic agent allows control on the biodistribution of drug, hence controlling the toxicity [12]. Nanoparticles allow drugs with lower molecular weight to stay in the circulation for a prolonged period [13]. Nanoparticles being 1000 times smaller than a cancer cell can easily cross the vasculature and reach the interstitium. Due to their small size, and a relatively large surface area allows loading with large number of molecules [14]. Nanoparticles also help to remove difficulties due to innate properties of active pharmaceutical ingredient (API) such as poor solubility can be overcome by using water-soluble polymers to trap the drug within [15]. Many chemotherapeutic agents which have low molecular weight face issue of hepatic clearance, but conversion into nanoparticles prevents quick clearance [16]. Nanoparticles reduce the exposure of drugs to the environment inside the body and prevent the degradation of the drugs and the side effects due to exposure of healthy cells to cytotoxic drugs [17]. Nanoparticles are being explored to give multiple actions at the same time. The researchers Xie et al. [18] inserted curcumin into nanoparticles made from bamboo charcoal. The nanoparticles were functionalized using D-α-tocopherol polyethylene glycol 1000 succinate. Due to a nano-formulation, the system gave better internalization, and this composite dosage form showed inhibition of P-gp which increased the efficacy of treatment. At the same time, the presence of antioxidants such as tocopherol and curcumin helped to remove any reactive radicals and showed radioprotective action [18]. Ma et al. [19] synthesized nanoparticles of poly-(acrylic acid) with CoSe using the aqueous precipitation method. These particles had photothermal transfer efficiency greater than 40% and negligible cytotoxicity. These nanoparticles were loaded with doxorubicin (DOX) which was shown to release in the acidic tumor conditions in cancer.

These particles gave a synergistic cytotoxic action due to chemotoxicity as well as phototoxicity [19].

Hu et al. [20] synthesized gold nanoparticles by rapidly reducing gold chloride trihydrate. To that solution, thio-PEG and thio-glucose were added which showed covalent bonding on gold nanoparticles. Glucose was attached to take advantage of excess glucose consumption of cancer cells as compared to normal body cells. The cells were allowed to take in the Glu-GNPs which were found to be effective than only irradiation or only gold nanoparticles [20].

3. Barriers to drug delivery in solid tumors

Tumors are a major presentation in cancer which exhibit presence of abnormal cellular and extracellular elements which can create obstacles in drug delivery to cancer cells situated deep within the tumors. Below given are barriers to drug delivery in tumors and ways to overcome those barriers-.

3.1 Biological barriers

Biological barriers include physiological components which prevent the reach of drug to tumors. To reach the desired site, the drug should circulate in the blood. Blood contains many proteins that form a structure around the drug particle called 'protein corona'. This phenomenon is called opsonization, and such opsonized particle is destroyed by phagocytes and macrophages. The physical characters of nanoparticle are determinants of extent of opsonization [21]. To prevent opsonization, the circulatory time is controlled using polymers such as PEG [22]. Yapa et al. targeted leucocytes and neural stem cells to facilitate entry into tumors as well as targeting metastases. The nanosponges were formulated using cholesterol and a CASPASE-6 sequence ((cholesterol-(K/D)nDEVDGC)3-trimaleimide) attached to a triangular maleimide linker which were then used to join lysine or aspartic acid. These function as apoptotic bodies and destroy the tumors [23]. If the nanoparticle avoids being opsonized, it still has to face many challenges to reach to its target sites, one being endothelium of blood vessels which is selectively permeable and on the top of that, being 'coated' by a negatively charged glycocalyx, it further restricts the reaction of particles with endothelial membrane [24]. Haemodynamic involves movement of nanoparticles through the blood vessels. As erythrocytes flow in the centre of the vessel, the other contents of blood are forced to move along the walls of the vessel. Understanding this phenomenon in context of nanoparticles will be helpful in design of better nanoparticles [25]. Particles larger than 5–6 nm are not able to squeeze through the continuous endothelium of a 'healthy' capillary. But in case of tumors, endothelial lining is more permeable and does not remain continuous. So, nanoparticles larger than 6 nm can cross these gaps to enter into the tumor microenvironment [26]. Because of inadequate lymphatic drainage, those particles do not get removed from the body. There is also a disparity in the sizes of the pores, which can be found in primary tumors, metastasized tumors, and even the same primary tumor, which is another drawback of this the enhanced permeability and retention effect (EPR) effect [27].

3.2 Tumor microenvironment

After the nanoparticle crosses successfully the endothelium and enters the tumor, it still has to cross the tortuous tumor microenvironment to reach to the tumor cells. The microenvironment consists of the tumor extracellular matrix that contains a network of collagen, elastin incorporating proteoglycans and hyaluronic acid. It maintains the tumor structure and provides nutrients and oxygen to cells. If the matrix is highly developed, it may cause the drug to get released far away from the target site [28]. Incorporating collagenase in the nanoparticles may help circumvent the collagen barrier and allow reach of nanoparticles [29]. The tumor growth cannot be infinite and is arrested because of presence of an extracellular matrix. The extracellular matrix also prevents efficient metastasis of the tumor cells. Tumor cells release various enzymes to degrade this matrix which are called matrix metalloproteinases [30]. These can be used in diagnosis of cancer as a marker. In this enzyme family, types 2 and 9 are more important in formation of tumors. Using drugs which inhibit metalloproteinases can be a best possible approach to counter this resistance [31]. Wang et al. synthesized nanosponges loaded with matrix metalloproteinase-14 inhibitor naphthofluorescein, which targets collagen in cardiovascular disease [32]. Flow of interstitial fluid in the tumor affects drug distribution as the drug exits vasculature from interstitium and finally reaches to cells. The movement occurs either by a concentration or a pressure gradient. As the blood vessel network is not uniform within a tumor, so the blood flow becomes uneven. Also, the drainage of interstitial fluid is poor due to poorly formed lymphatic network. It increases the interstitial fluid pressure. Due to high heterogeneity in tumor structure, the fluid pressure can be different for two tumors in the same organism [33]. As cancer cells prefer a type of fermentation over aerobic respiration, the amount of oxygen decreases and the number of acids increases near the centre. These conditions make the tumor resistant to certain treatments as radiation [34]. Hypoxia causes increased production of chemokines which promote angiogenesis and avoids detection from immune cells [35]. Also, the acidic pH may aid in targeting by using acid-sensitive polymers to release medication at the centre of tumor [36]. Caldera et al. synthesized nanosponges from cyclic nigerosyl-1-6 nigerose using pyromellitic dianhydride as a crosslinker. The nanosponges were prepared using high-pressure homogenization and showed swelling at lower pH which caused DOX release [37].

3.3 Cellular barriers

Cellular barriers include various cellular components which prevent the reach of the drug to intracellular environment. Many drugs show their effects inside the cell. Hence, even if the drug reaches near cancer cells inside the tumor, it has to cross the cell membrane to enter inside the cell to exert its actions. The carrier should interact with cell membrane to achieve the release [38]. Physical characteristics of carrier such as size, surface charge and hydrophobicity affect the interaction with cell membrane. Charged particles show more interaction with cell membrane. Neutral particles may crowd near cell membrane preventing any further entry into the cell [39]. Particles smaller than 200 nm get internalized by clathrin-mediated endocytosis, and those which are larger undergo clavioline-mediated endocytosis. This process is an energy-dependent process. Cancer cell membranes express many ligands which can be targeted [40]. Singh et al. [41] prepared cyclodextrin nanosponges and attached cholesterol as a functionalization moiety. Cholesterol being a major component of cell membrane facilitates easy interactions with cell membrane and hence easy penetration in cells.

3.4 Organellar and vesicular barriers

Once inside the cell, the carrier should travel to the designated target site so as to release the drug. This travel is mediated by endosomes, which is energy-dependent. Endocytosis occurs by various pathways physiologically, and the pathways may be different for different types of nanoparticles. Generally, all these pathways end up in taking contents to lysosomes where they are destroyed. Use of fusogenic lipids is advised to prevent this fate [42]. Yan et al. synthesized nanosponges and coated them with fusogenic lipids which enhanced internalization and a better delivery inside the cells [43].

3.5 Drug efflux transporters

Till the medications reach the target site, only a small fraction of original dose remains which shows its effect. Hence, many tumors contain efflux pumps which remove the drugs out of tumor cells [44]. P-glycoprotein is one such receptor to throw the drugs out of cells. Various small molecules which are P-glycoprotein inhibitors can be used to avoid the efflux [45]. Arima et al. [46] prepared nanosponges of dimethyl-β-cyclodextrin and loaded them with an immunosuppressant tacrolimus. These complexes were tested on rats where they showed increased bioavailability and dissolution rate. Pre-treatment of apical membrane with dimethyl-β-cyclodextrin showed dislodging of receptors from the membrane and successfully inhibited P-glycoprotein showing increased absorption of drugs [46].

4. Definition of nanosponges

Nanosponges are sponges of very small size with diameter less than 1 μm. These are three-dimensional networks made of polymers which act as frames to hold the drug molecules inside them. These sponges circulate the body and can release the drug at a specific site [47].

4.1 Advantages of nanosponge

Nanosponges offer advantages over other nanoparticles such as a targeted release of active constituents inside the body which is caused due to functionalization on the surface. Nanosponges allow flexibility of formulation due to various polymers used as well as stability due to the drug entering the pores of sponge. These are non-toxic, non-allergenic and non-mutagenic due to biocompatible ingredients used. As these sponges are made of biodegradable molecules, they are able to provide extended release due to slow degradation of drug. Nanosponges are stable over wide temperature range and show excellent stability over the pH range. As nanosponges have diameter less than a bacterium, the formulation is self-sterile as bacteria are unable to enter the formulation. They exhibit excellent thermal, physical and chemical stability [48].

4.2 Disadvantages of nanosponge

Nanosponges can be used for only small molecules as large molecules may not enter the nanosized pores of nanosponge. The drug loading is also affected by the degree of crystallization. Dose dumping may be observed due to sudden degradation of carrier [49].

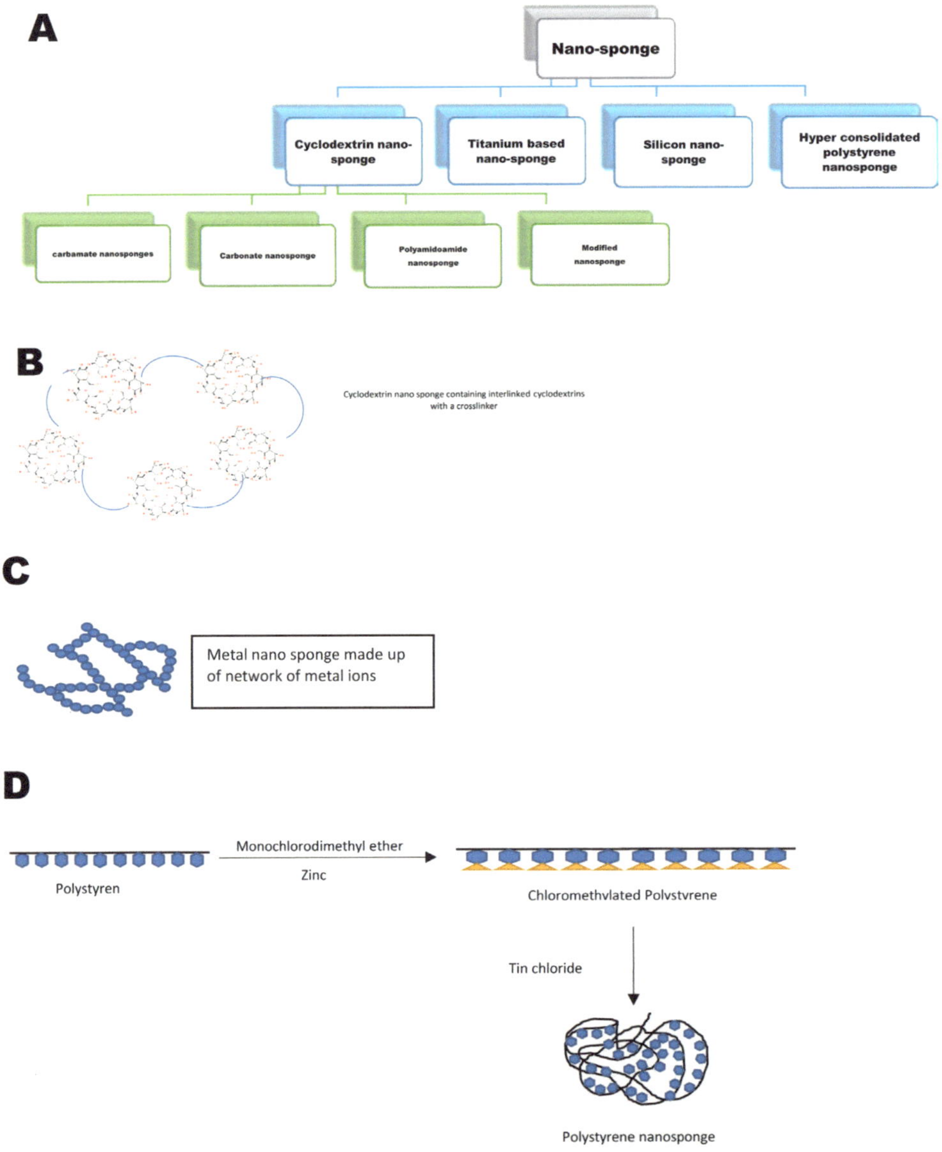

Figure 1.
(A) Classification of nanosponge—this figure shows classification of nanosponges based on the materials used for synthesis. (B) Beta-cyclodextrin nanosponge—beta-cyclodextrin nanosponges are prepared by crosslinking beta-cyclodextrin molecules using crosslinkers. (C) Metal nanosponge—these are made by irregular arrangements of metal nanoparticles in irregular ways to create pores and channels on the surface. (D) Polystyrene nanosponge—the polystyrene is chloromethylated and reacted with tin chloride to give a hyper-condensed polymeric nanosponge.

5. Classification of nanosponges

The classification of nanosponges based on the material used is illustrated in **Figure 1A** [50].

Type	Crosslinker used	Example	Method used
Cyclodextrin carbonate nanosponges	Carbonyl crosslinkers	Diphenyl carbonate Dimethyl carbonate	Thermal deposition Solvent extraction
Cyclodextrin carbamate nanosponges	Diisocyanate crosslinkers	Hexamethylene diisocyanate Toluene diisocyanate	Solvent method
Cyclodextrin anhydride nanosponges	Anhydride crosslinkers	Pyromellitic dianhydride EDTA dianhydride	Solvent method
Epichlorohydrin cyclodextrin nanosponges	Epichlorohydrin crosslinkers	Epichlorohydrin	Solvent method

Table 1.
Different types of beta-cyclodextrin-based nanosponges.

5.1 Cyclodextrin-based nanosponges

Cyclodextrins have been majorly used for the preparation of nanosponges. These are cyclic oligosaccharides. These are cone-shaped molecules made of glucopyranose units. These units are arranged around a hydrophobic hollow core which is used to trap any molecules.

Selection of crosslinkers is important to alter the properties of the final product. Crosslinkers such as epichlorohydrin give cyclodextrin nanosponges with hydrophilic pores whereas crosslinkers such as diphenyl carbonate and diisocyanates give hydrophobic nanosponges [51]. Various types of cyclodextrin-based nanosponges are enlisted in **Table 1** and **Figure 1B** [52].

5.2 Metal and metal oxide nanosponges

Metal and metal oxide nanosponges have desirable characters such as a wide surface area, small particle size and better stability. Metal oxides are being shown interest due to their ability of interaction with other species such as atoms, ions and molecules. They are able to form a porous interconnected network and show properties different than bulk. These also show magnetism and semiconductor properties. Metallic nanosponges can be made from one, two or multiple metals simultaneously. The nanosponges made from two or more metals are desirable over those made from single metal as they are more porous and based on porosity, and they can be classified as micro, meso and microporous based on the size of sponge where microporous are smaller than 2 nm, macroporous being larger than 50 nm and mesoporous lying in between them (**Figure 1C**) [53].

5.3 Polystyrene nanosponges

Davankov et al. [54] prepared nanosponges of linear polystyrene by causing intramolecular hyper-crosslinking. The polymer was initially chloromethylated using dichloro monoethyl ether, and this solution was added to the solution of zinc chloride in the same ether which acted as a catalyst. This mixture was heated at 40°C for 3 h. The precipitated polymer was washed and dried. This polymer is dissolved in 2 L ethylene dichloride distilled over phosphorous pentoxide. Tin chloride solution was added which changed the colors gradually from pink to brown. Acetone was added to dissolve colored complex. The solution was allowed to cool and was washed with water. The organic layer was separated and concentrated to 20% of starting volume. The nanosponges were isolated using methanol. They were dried and stored (**Figure 1D**) [54].

6. Mechanism and preparation of polymeric nanosponges

For the formation of nanosponges made out of polymer, reaction conditions such as heat and solvents promote uncoiling of long polymer chains and reveal the groups for reaction with crosslinkers. Crosslinkers such as diphenyl carbonate release the phenyl group upon reaction which remains in reaction mixture, and the carbonyl group acts as crosslinkers during the formation of nanosponges. The extensive crosslinking causes winding and coiling of long polymer chains and forms pores and cavities leading to the formation of nanosponges. The prepared formulation is later purified using organic solvents such as ethanol to remove those impurities.

6.1 Melt method

Cyclodextrins are made to react with crosslinkers like diphenyl carbonate, dimethyl carbonate and diisocyanates. All the dry ingredients are homogenously mixed and put into a flask and heated at 100°C. A magnetic stirrer is used to achieve uniform mixing of contents. The heating is kept up for a total of 5 h so that the reaction can take place. After allowing the mixture to cool down, the obtained solid is broken up into smaller pieces using mortar. It is then purified using the Soxhlet extraction method after being washed to remove any unreacted reactants [55]. Sadjadi et al. synthesized beta-cyclodextrin nanosponges using the melt method. A calculated amount of diphenyl carbonate was melted at 90°C in a beaker. Preheated beta-cyclodextrin was added to it. The mixture was stirred for half a day at temperature exceeding 100°C to allow reaction to get completed. The solidified product was cooled and pulverized. The product was washed using water and organic solvent and later purified using Soxhlet extraction [56].

6.2 Solvent diffusion method

6.2.1 Emulsion solvent diffusion method

Ethyl cellulose and polyvinyl alcohol are used to prepare nanosponges. Cellulose and drug are dissolved in organic solvent such as dichloromethane. Then this dispersed phase is added to continuous phase which is aqueous poly (vinyl) alcohol (PVA) solution. This mixture is stirred at high speed for a specific amount of time, and the product is filtered and dried [57]. Solunke et al. [58] prepared gliclazide nanosponges using emulsion solvent diffusion method. Gliclazide and Eudragit were added to organic phase, and aqueous phase was a PVA solution. Organic phase was added to aqueous phase, it was stirred, and nanosponges were collected and washed [58].

6.2.2 Quasi-emulsion solvent diffusion

This process involves polymers such as Eudragit. The polymer is dissolved into a solvent and the drug is added to same solution. This inner phase is added to PVA solution and stirred. The product is filtered out and dried [59]. Salunke et al. [60] prepared budesonide-loaded nanosponges by quasi-emulsion solvent diffusion method. Weighed amounts of Polymethyl-methacrylate (PMMA) and Eudragit S-100 were dissolved in organic solvent containing dichloromethane and methanol in equal proportions. Dibutyl phthalate was added to enhance polymer plasticity. The organic phase was added to aqueous PVA solution and was stirred for 2 h. The prepared nanosponges were recovered by filtration and were washed and dried [60].

6.3 Solvent method

The polymer is mixed with an aprotic solvent such as dimethyl sulfoxide. Carbonyl crosslinkers are added to this solution. The reaction is allowed to take place at a range of temperature which may not increase the boiling point of solvent. The solution is cooled at room temperature, and a large amount of water is added to it. The product is recovered by filtration [61]. Rao et al. [62] synthesized nanosponges by the solvent method by dissolving anhydrous β-cyclodextrin and diphenyl carbonate and heating that solution at 90–100°C under stirring. The prepared product was washed with water and later with organic solvents to remove any unreacted constituents. The product was dried to use later [62].

6.4 Ultrasound assisted synthesis

This method involves energy from ultrasound to carry on the reaction. The reactants are placed in the flask and heated with help of ultrasound. The mixture is allowed to react. Later the product is cooled down and broken with mortar. The product is washed with water and purified by Soxhlet apparatus [63]. Jasim et al. [63] prepared cyclodextrin nanosponges using ultrasound-assisted method. Weighed quantities of β-CD and diphenyl carbonate. The mixture was heated on an oil bath and was sonicated using a probe sonicator at 50% amplitude for 4 h. The product was broken down and washed to give final product [63].

7. Mechanism and methods of metal and metal oxide nanosponge formation

Metal nanosponges are prepared by reducing a metal salt using a suitable reagent. Surfactants or capping agents are used to control the growth rate and structure of nanosponges. Ghosh and Jagirdar [64] prepared silver nanosponges in their research activity. Silver nitrate was used as a substrate for synthesis on nanosponge. The salt was reduced to silver cations using boranes. This reaction was carried out at a temperature above 300 K. The reduced metal salt releases free metal atoms. These join together to form nanoparticles. These nanoparticles join together to form nanosponges due to their irregular joining which produce pores or gaps in the structure. This process works like bottom-up approach of synthesis of nanoparticles as they are built from the atoms themselves [64]. Different mechanisms are used to prepare metal oxide nanosponges such as precipitation and removal from alloy. Dealloying involves removal of a more reactive metal from an alloy. Chemical dealloying is the most common method involving use of acids to react with more reactive metal to remove it from the alloy. Alloy nature and leaching conditions affect this process. Another method utilizes the mechanism of precipitation of metal separated from its salt. This separation is brought about by using reducing agents such as $NaBH_4$. Later, it is heated at very high temperature to deposit the metal oxide which gives out hydrogen bubbles which are responsible for generation of channels and pores which are required for drug loading. A disadvantage is the variable pore size due to uncontrolled particle size which gets sedimented. Electrochemical deposition utilizes the mechanism of movement of ions towards the oppositely charged electrodes. The ions that migrate form a thin film on the surface of metallic/metal electrode. The changes in pH, temperature and current density can be carried out to vary the properties of the sponge prepared. Another method based on hydrolysis of metal precursors and their conversion to metal species is the sol-gel method. It involves electrolysis of metal compounds in 'sol' phase in a solvent. After passing the electric current, the metal particles deposit on the electrode with internal pores and cavities in form of gel. The coagulation of prepared particles can be avoided by altering pH of medium. Drying is performed by evaporation or supercritical methods which evaporate the solvent and forms pores [53].

8. Advantages of nanosponges over other nanocarriers

Nanoparticles after reaching the site of action release their loaded drug all at once creating a 'burst'. Hence, effective dosage cannot be determined properly, whereas nanoparticles being made of biodegradable polymers release their drugs in a slow, controlled manner after the sponges encounter a tumor [48]. Nanosponges are soluble in aqueous as well as organic solvents. These are non-toxic carriers which are heat-stable [65]. Nanosponges are water-soluble which allow the researchers to use them for dissolution of insoluble drugs after loading them into the sponge [66]. Loading and functionalization of nanosponges is pretty easy as compared to other nanoparticles. The functional groups protruding out of nanosponge surface can be used for post-modification strategies such as functionalization [67]. Many nanoparticles have complex chemistry; hence, they cannot be scaled up easily for large-scale production. On the other hand, nanosponges made of only polymers and crosslinkers are easy to scale up for commercial production [68]. As compared to other nanoparticles, where reconstruction of nanoparticles is difficult if they lose their structure, nanosponges can be easily remade by methods such as washing with eco-compatible solvents, mild heating or changing pH or ionic strength [69]. Where many types of nanoparticles are used to contain solid medications, nanosponges can be used to encapsulate not only solids but also liquids and gaseous drugs [70]. Nanosponges can be used to load both hydrophilic and hydrophobic drugs owing to the hydrophobic core and external hydrophilic branching. Hence, these nanostructures can be flexibly loaded with hydrophilic or hydrophobic molecules [71]. **Figure 2** highlights major researches on nanosponges from 2005 to 2022.

9. Methods of preparation of nanosponges

Nanosponges can be prepared with a variety of methods and then can be loaded to give a varying amount of drug loading. Kumar et al. [72] prepared cyclodextrin

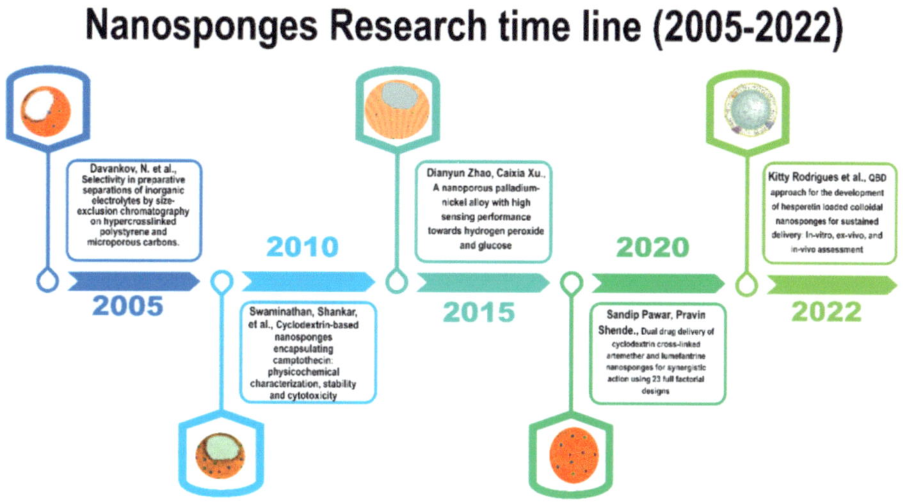

Figure 2.
Nanosponges major research timeline.

nanosponges loaded with babchi oil using tiring at high speed. Similar approaches are described in **Table 2.**

10. Optimization of nanosponges

Optimization involves obtaining a best combination of starting materials to get a formula which gives the desired results. Due to a simple composition, nanosponges can be optimized without much hassle, which is evident from the examples given in **Table 3**.

11. Morphological characterization

Morphological characterization involves various instrumental methods to analyze the morphology of prepared nanostructure. Transmission electron microscopy (TEM) involves scanning a sample with a beam of focused electrons which is transmitted through the sample to understand composition of particle. Argenziano et al. [86] prepared β-cyclodextrin nanosponges loaded with paclitaxel. Pyromellitic anhydride was used as a crosslinking agent. Methods such as high-pressure homogenization were used to reduce the particle size. The analysis was performed on Philips CM 10 device. The sample was prepared on formvar-coated copper. The coated samples were air-dried. The results showed that spherical particles were formed. The size was in nano-range due to application of high-pressure homogenization in the synthesis of nanosponges [86]. Scanning electron microscopy involves scanning a sample using an electron beam focused on sample which is then converted into signals. Mady and Mohamed Ibrahim (2018) prepared nanosponges using β-cyclodextrin and diphenyl carbonate crosslinker in DMF as solvent. The mixture was sonicated and refluxed using water and ethanol to remove impurities. Scanning electron microscopy was carried out using model LEO-435 VP, Cambridge (UK). It was used at 15 KV accelerating

Polymer	Drug	Loading method	Loading efficiency	Reference
B-Cyclodextrin	Babchi oil	Blank NS were dispersed in water. Excess amount of babchi oil was added and stirred for 24 h. The suspension was centrifuged. The supernatant was freeze-dried	21.47% w/w maximum and 14.23% minimum	[72]
β-Cyclodextrin	Griseofulvin	Drug dispersed in aqueous colloidal dispersion of NS having PVP. Suspension was stirred and centrifuged. Supernatant was freeze-dried	Maximum 47.2% and minimum 20.20%, based on formation of ternary complex	[73]
β-Cyclodextrin	Celecoxib	Method 1: Drug and polymer were dissolved in dimethyl formamide. This solution was stirred. Crosslinker was added to same solution. (internal phase) This was added to water (external phase) and stirred. The suspension was lyophilized	After using N,N-methylene bisacrylamide, 22.11 ± 0.41 to 26.26 ± 0.24%. Loading was seen.	[74]
		Method 2: Drug and polymer were dissolved in dimethyl formamide. (internal phase) This was added to crosslinker in water (external phase) and stirred. The dispersion was lyophilized	After using glyoxal, 22.48 ± 0.23 to 24.85 ± 0.47% loading was achieved	
B-Cyclodextrin	Piperine	NS were suspended in water and stirred. Then the drug is gradually added. The dispersion was sonicated and then stirred. The suspension was centrifuged to remove excess of drug. The supernatant was lyophilized and stored in a desiccator.	Loading efficiency was 42.6 ± 1.1%	[75]
B-Cyclodextrin in Fe_3O_4 nanoparticles coated by β-CD NS	Curcumin	Nanoparticles were dispersed in PBS. Curcumin solution in acetone was added to the suspension. Mixture was shaken overnight in dark. The product was separated using a magnet and washed by de-ionized water	Loading efficiency was 96% at 1:2 ratio of drug: carrier	[76]

B-Cyclodextrin	Camptothecin	Drug was added to aqueous nanosponge suspension and stirred for 24 h in dark. The suspension was centrifuged to separate free drug. Colloidal supernatant was freeze-dried	Loading efficiency was 38% w/w	[77]
B-Cyclodextrin	Curcumin	Curcumin dissolved in dichloromethane. Nanosponges were added to this solution and triturated till solvent evaporates. The product was dried	46.45 ± 0.54 mg and 48.37 ± 0.47 mg of curcumin/100 mg of F1 and F2 respectively	[78]
B-Cyclodextrin	Nifedipine	Prepared nanosponges and nifedipine in excess were mixed and were suspended in distilled water. The mixture was sonicated and then stirred. Aq. Suspension centrifuged to separate free drug. Supernatant was lyophilized	Encapsulation efficiency was 78.4 ± 0.24%	[79]
Ethyl cellulose	Lansoprazole	Drug and polymer were added to dichloromethane. This disperse phase was added to aq. PVA solution. Mixture stirred for 2 h. Prepared NS were filtered and dried	Entrapment efficiency was 86.93 ± 0.65% in F2	[80]

Table 2.
Methods of preparation of nanosponges.

voltage, and different resolutions were used to obtain images. The images showed a perfect spherical shape of loaded nanosponges. Some drug particles were present on the surface as well as numerous porous channels were present on the surface. As compared to blank nanosponges, drug-loaded nanosponges were more porous [87]. Atomic force microscopy involves interactions of probe with sample through up-down and side-to-side movement along area of sample which is checked using a laser beam. Choudhary et al. [88] synthesized two peptides. And these linked peptides were attached to a trimaleimide frame. It gave two structures with positive and negative charge. Then using those differently charged structures, two variants were formed having 15 and 20 subunits, respectively. These two types of structures were mixed under conditions mimicking human body which resulted in the formation of nanosponges. 0.05 M stock solution of NS was prepared in PBS, and a drop was added on a freshly prepared mica sheet. The buffer was removed using nitrogen stream for 2 min. Bruker Innova AFM system was used to take the pictures using a TESPA-HAR probe in tapping mode. Spring constant was kept 50 N/m and operated at a frequency of 350 KHz. Images were taken at a scan rate of 1 Hz. The structures with 15 subunits showed formation of bundles made from three to five subunits. The structure with 20 subunits formed excellent nanosponges in the range of 80–115 nm [88].

Sr. no.	Model used	Dependent var.	Results	Reference
1	Box-Behnken	Polymer conc (mol) Crosslinker conc (mol) Reaction time Particle size Entrapment efficiency	Particle size depends directly on polymer concentration	[81]
2	3^2 full factorial design	Amt of β-CD (gm) Amt of DPC (gm) Porosity Zeta potential Drug loading Drug release	As B-CD conc increase and porosity increases. Zeta potential depends on particle size only. Drug loading depends upon DPC conc.	[82]
3	3^2 full factorial design	THCL:EC ratio (w/w) Stirring rate (rpm) Particle size Production yield (%) Entrapment efficiency	Particle size reduced as stirring rate increased. Entrapment efficiency decreased by increasing stirring rate. Production yield increases as polymer conc increases.	[83]
4	Robust model	Amount of EC Amount of PVA Particle size Entrapment efficiency	Particle size increases with increase in drug-polymer ratio.	[84]
5	2^3 full factorial design	Amount of HP-β Amount of β-CD Amount of CDI % Entrapment efficiency Particle size	Particle size decreases with increase in concentration of CDI and β-CD. % Entrapment efficiency increases with increase in concentration of HPβ-CD and β-CD.	[85]

Table 3.
Optimization of nanosponges.

Photon correlation spectroscopy involves measuring Brownian motion of particles as a function of time which is recorded by scattering of laser where scattering is directly proportional to particle size. Yakavets et al. [89] synthesized nanosponges from ethyl cellulose, PVA and pleuronic F68 by emulsion solvent diffusion technique. The particle size was measured using a Nano ZS-90 (Malvern instruments Ltd., UK) at an angle of 25°. The sample was diluted 10 times and analyzed. The composition F2 showed minimum particle size at 83 nm [89]. Wang and Schaaf [90] synthesized size-controlled Au-Ag nanosponges. Their structural characterization was carried out using SEM and TEM. Advanced techniques, such as focused ion beam, were used to reveal the hybrid composition of nanosponges. 3D structural properties were analyzed using techniques such as synchrotron X-ray nanometography. Atom probe tomography can be used where the obtained images are aligned again and again to allow reconstruction of particle image and thus to obtain the parameters. Nanosponges have peculiar optical properties due to their complex structure. Properties such as optical scattering and photoluminescence can be measured using dark field florescence confocal microscopy [90]. The analytical techniques may vary with use of the final product. Maity et al. [91] synthesized nanosponges of acidic aminosilicates for the purpose of catalysis. Those were analyzed using morphological characterization techniques such as SEM and TEM which confirmed the formation of nanosponges as well as their porous structure. X-ray diffraction studies were carried out to understand the percentage of aluminium precursors. 1-D and 2-D NMR studies were carried out to understand the locations of catalytically active sites of nanosponges. A temperature-programmed desorption study using ammonia was carried out to understand the distribution of acidic sites in nanosponges and to identify their correlation with NMR data [91].

12. Encapsulation efficiency

Encapsulation efficiency indicates the amount of drug which gets successfully entrapped in a nanoparticle. Rezaei et al. (2019) prepared cyclodextrin nanosponges loaded with ferulic acid where three ratios of β-CD: crosslinker taken namely 1:2, 1:4 and 1:8 were synthesized. To determine the encapsulation efficiency, drug-loaded and blank nanosponges were suspended in ethanol and sonicated at room temperature separately. The sonicated dispersions were filtered using a filter paper with pore size of 0.45 μm. Ferulic acid content was determined using UV-visible spectrophotometry at 319 nm. The analysis showed that nanosponge prepared with 1:4 ratio of β-CD to crosslinker showed maximum encapsulation as lower ratio resulted in an insufficient amount of crosslinking and a ratio of 1:8 showed hyper-crosslinking, hence reducing the amount of encapsulated ferulic acid [92]. Dhakar et al. [93] prepared cyclodextrin nanosponges loaded with resveratrol and oxyresveratrol. The prepared nanosponges were added to water to give a solution of 10 mg/ml, and drugs were added in different ratios of drug: nanosponge, i.e. 1:2, 1:4 and 1:6. The mixtures were stirred for a day in dark after sonicating them for some time. The supernatant was collected after centrifugation of formulation, and it was lyophilized to give a dry powder. The powder was subjected to High-performance liquid chromatography(HPLC) analysis to understand loading of the drugs. The powder was taken in vials containing ethanol and sonicated for an hour. It was analyzed using High-performance liquid chromatography(HPLC). The drug loading was maximum in the ratio of drug to nanosponge which is 1:4, since saturation solubility was achieved. The encapsulation efficiency of the nanosponges was found to be 77% for resveratrol and 80% for oxyresveratrol. In addition, the encapsulation demonstrated an increase in the solubility of previously insoluble compounds. Diphenyl carbonate and beta-cyclodextrin were used to make nanosponges in various molar ratios, including 1:2, 1:4, 1:6, 1:8, and 1:10. Through the process of freeze-drying, which involved adding specific amounts of blank nanoparticles and babchi oil to water, stirring, and sonicating for a day, they were loaded with the babchi oil. The mixture was centrifuged to remove the oil which did not enter the inclusion complex. The supernatant was removed and freeze-dried. A specific amount of NS were added to dimethyl sulfoxide and sonicated to separate drugs from complex. The samples were analyzed using UV spectrophotometer at 265 nm. The encapsulation efficiency was observed in the range 62–93%. The maximum efficiency was present in formulation with the molar ratio of cyclodextrin to carrier 1:4. In formulations with higher number of crosslinking agents, hyper-crosslinking resulted in less loading [72]. Appleton et al. [94] prepared β-cyclodextrin nanosponges by reacting polymer, triethanolamine and pyromellitic dianhydride in DMSO at 90° in an RBF. The prepared product was solidified, washed and ground. The coarse product was ground and purified with acetone using Soxhlet extraction. Insulin was loaded in blank carriers by mixing an acidic solution of drug in a solution of nano-formulation where the ratio between insulin and nanosponges was 1:5. The mixture was stirred, and the sediment was lyophilized. Such prepared nanosponges were added to a mobile phase in a proper concentration and sonicated. The solvent was analyzed using UV spectrophotometry. The encapsulation efficiency was 91% [94]. The product was washed using water and ethanol and later purified using Soxhlet extraction. For loading, solvents such as ethanol, methanol, acetone and only essential oil were tested for four different time intervals from 1 to 4 days. A weighed quantity of nanosponges were placed in a microtube, and coriander essential oil dissolved in a solvent was added. The mixture was stirred at room temperature to facilitate loading. Then the sample was centrifuged to separate the loaded nanosponges and was freeze-dried. After freeze-drying, the samples were dispersed in acetone and stirred for a day which were later centrifuged to separate the acetone supernatant. The obtained supernatants were analyzed using Gas chromatography–mass spectrometry (GC-MS). Five major constituents such as pinene, cynene, camphor, linalool and geranyl acetate were used to detect quantitatively [95].

13. Nanosponges for delivery of anticancer drug

Anticancer drugs are notoriously famous for their side effects which can be decreased by the use of nano-formulations which reduce the dose required and hence the side effects. Wang et al. synthesized nanosponges from DNAzyme-containing ZnO to release therapeutically active ROS [96]. **Table 4** indicates such similar results and show enhanced action of dosage forms over administration of single API.

14. Functionalization of nanosponges

Functionalization involves attachment of various functional group or functional molecules on nanoparticle surface. Such a process imparts targeting properties to the nanoparticle. Femminò et al. functionalized cyclodextrin nanosponges using oxygen to relieve hypoxic conditions in ailments such as tumors [103]. Some examples of functionalization of nanosponges using chemical as well as biological functional ingredients are shown in **Table 5.**

15. Future trends

Nanosponges have been limited for catalytic action or use as a carrier. Mostly simple nanosponges or those with basic functionalization are synthesized and used for delivery of single therapeutic agents, but the future trends are nanosponges that have been designed for storage of phase change materials. 3-D carbon-based materials such as nanosponges are preferred for loading of phase change materials which can be applied in locations such as operation tables, storage of medical and pharmaceutical products. Nanosponges can show advantages for application of both solid- and liquid-phase change

Drug	Polymer	Cancer type	Studies performed	Results	References
Doxorubicin	B-cyclodextrin	Breast cancer	Human MDA-MB231 and MCF-7 cell lines, mouse 4T1 (DOX-sensitive) and EMT6/AR10r (DOX-resistant) cell lines, efficacy using MTT assay	Concentration-dependent inhibition of cell viability which was more than doxorubicin	[97]
Erlotinib	B-cyclodextrin conjugated with glutathione	Lung cancer	Human lung carcinoma cells (A549 cells), MTT assay to determine efficacy	Dose- and time-dependent inhibition of proliferation of A549 cells. Nanosponges showed better effect at lower dose than only erlotinib.	[98]
Paclitaxel	B-cyclodextrin	Melanoma	Types of human cell lines used—A375, M14, JR8, RPMI7932, PCF-2 and LM. Types of mice cell lines used—B16-BL6	The formulation showed increased oral bioavailability and efficacy as compared to free drug. The formulation showed considerably lesser toxicity as compared to free drug. The formulation also showed inhibition of metastasis and growth.	[99]
Ferulic acid	B-cyclodextrin	Breast cancer	MCF7 cell lines for human breast cancer and 4T1 cell line for mouse breast cancer, using MTT assay	The cytotoxicity was observed at concentration above 500 μM. The cytotoxic effect was time-dependent. As the formulation enhanced the solubility, the inhibitory concentration was reduced.	[92]
Strigolactone	B-cyclodextrin conjugated with glutathione	Prostate cancer	DU145 and PC-3 prostate cancer cells, efficiency studied using MTT assay	The free drug as well as nanosponges inhibited the cell proliferation. This activity on the formulation was dependent on intracellular GSH amount.	[100]
Bortezomib	B-cyclodextrin	Breast cancer	MCF-7 cell lines for human breast cancer were used, and MTT assay for checking the proliferation	The complex showed high loading, sustained release, and aqueous dispersion. The cytotoxicity was found to be reduced due to sustained release effect	[101]

Drug	Polymer	Cancer type	Studies performed	Results	References
Naphthofluorescein	Poly(VL-AVL-EVL) conjugated with T-Peptide_ACPP and cyanine-3 hydrazide		RAW cells and HT1080 cells were used; MTT assay used for testing efficacy	The formulation was able to locate collagen in presence of MMP2 enzyme. Both the types of cells showed a good extent of internalization.	[32]
Doxorubicin	Oligonucleotide DNA		MCF-7 cells and Hs 578 Bst cells were used for analysis, and MTT assay used for efficiency	The DNA nanosponges were broken down at acidic pH. These carriers were able to overcome barriers and target cells. The cytotoxicity was similar to free drug due to less release	[102]

Table 4.
Nanosponges for delivery of anticancer drugs.

Polymer	Functionalized by	Rationale	Reference
PLGA	Cancer cell membrane	By coating with cancer cell membrane, the particle shows homologous binding and bio-mimetic and targeting capacity. It possesses properties of a cancer cell to allow targeting.	[104]
Carbon quantum dot-polyethylene glycol bisacrylate	Hydrazine	The carboxyl groups of Crosslinked carbon quantum dots (CQDs) were amidated using hydrazine to imine to give an acid labile bond which will be broken down in acidic tumor environment.	[105]
Fe_3O_4 nanoparticles coated with B-CD nanosponge	Folic acid	Fe_3O_4 nanoparticles as a core to provide clear visualization during MRI. Folic acid for smart drug delivery and specific targeting.	[78]
B-cyclodextrin	Cholesterol	Cholesterol is a major component of cell membrane. Attachment of cholesterol on surface of nanosponges allows bioadhesion and enhances cellular uptake.	[41]
Gold nanosponge	Poly (N-isopropylacrylamide–methacrylic acid–1,4-dioxane, octadecyl acrylate)	pH- and thermal-responsive polymer.	[106]
	EpDT3	An aptamer which binds to EpCAM, a biomarker present on cancer cell, helps on targeting.	
Reduced graphene oxide-lipid nanosponge	Protein Lf (Lactoferrin)	Lactoferrin shows selectivity towards cancer cell and inhibits cancer cell proliferation and migration.	[107]

Table 5.
Functionalization of nanosponges.

materials. Carbon nanosponges have high loading and can be filled with a high number of materials. And nanosponges do not behave to changes in temperature [108–110]. Korea Ceramic Technology Institute developed a thermosponge for the treatment of cancer. It is a thermoresponsive nanosponge used for delivery of both hydrophilic and hydrophobic drugs. This nanosponge is made up of a core of poly-D, L-lactide which is loaded with a hydrophobic drug and the outer covering is made up of Pluronic-F127 which is loaded with a hydrophilic drug. The drugs can be released at the same time or the drug entrapped in the core may be released at a later time showing a prolonged release. The system is biodegradable and biocompatible, hence showing very less to no toxicity at all.

16. Conclusion

In this review, nanosponges and their synthesis, characterization, optimization and applications regarding cancer have been discussed. According to the literature, nanosponges can be classified based on their starting materials which could be polymers, metals, metal oxides, etc. Polymer nanosponges can be manufactured by methods such as melt method, emulsion method, solvent method and ultrasound-assisted method. Metallic nanosponges are manufactured by methods such as dealloying and sol-gel methods. Factors related to drugs or process parameters influence formation of nanosponges. These process parameters were used by many researchers to optimize the formulation of nanosponges to give the optimum results related to loading efficiency, particle size and encapsulation efficiency. Polymer structure also affects the formation of nanosponges. Tumors are important manifestations of cancer and provide many challenges to deliver drugs inside the tumor where dividing cells are located. These challenges can be overcome by the process of functionalization with chemical moieties or biological entities such as cell membrane fragments. Such prepared nanosponges can be characterized with many methods such as SEM and TEM which are reported in literature. Toxicity of nanosponges may be a growing concern due to their ever-increasing role in multiple industries. According to the literature, nanosponges are safe for use as a carrier. But their nanosize may alter their properties, and hence reactivity causes toxicity due to processes such as physical interaction, ROS generation and intracellular dissolution. Many methods have been reported in literature such as using antioxidants and altering the material available to reduce this toxicity.

Declaration of interest statement

Authors declare there are no conflicts of interest.

Abbreviations

CD	cyclodextrin
NS	nanosponges
PVA	poly (vinyl) alcohol
PBS	phosphate buffer saline
EC	ethyl cellulose
DMF	dimethyl formamide
PEG	poly (ethylene) glycol
HP-β	hydroxypropyl beta cyclodextrin
API	active pharmaceutical ingredient
P-gp	P-glycoprotein
DOX	doxorubicin
DNA	deoxy ribonucleic acid

Author details

Kapil Gore[1], Sankha Bhattacharya[1] and Bhupendra Prajapati[2*]

1 Department of Pharmaceutics, School of Pharmacy and Technology Management, SVKM'S NMIMS Deemed-to-be University, Shirpur, Maharashtra, India

2 Shree S.K. Patel College of Pharmaceutical Education and Research, Ganpat University, Gujarat, India

*Address all correspondence to: bhupendra.prajapati@ganpatuniversity.ac.in, bhupen27@gmail.com

References

[1] Yadav AR, Mohite SK. Cancer—A silent killer: An overview. Asian Journal of Pharmaceutical Research. 2020;**10**(3):213-216

[2] Steeg PS. Targeting metastasis. Nature Reviews Cancer. 2016;**16**(4): 201-218

[3] Organization WH. Noncommunicable diseases country profiles 2018. 2018

[4] Abbas Z, Rehman S. An overview of cancer treatment modalities. Neoplasm 1. London: IntechOpen; 2018:139-157

[5] Zugazagoitia J et al. Current challenges in cancer treatment. Clinical Therapeutics. 2016;**38**(7):1551-1566

[6] Saltzstein HC. Possibilities and limitations of surgery in cancer; a follow-up study of 572 personally treated patients. Harper Hospital Bulletin. 1956;**14**(5):297-305

[7] Bhattacharya S, Sharma P, Mathur H, Rasheed H, Singh S, Rajput G, et al. Recent apprise on coronavirus and its terrible insinuations. VirusDisease. 2020;**31**:121-127

[8] Hussain Z, Khan JA, Murtaza S. Nanotechnology: An Emerging Therapeutic Option for Breast Cancer. Critical Reviews in Eukaryotic Gene Expression. 2018;**28**(2):163-175. DOI: 10.1615/CritRevEukaryotGeneExpr.2018022771. PMID: 30055543

[9] Bhattacharya S, Saindane D, Prajapati BG. Liposomal Drug Delivery And Its Potential Impact On Cancer Research. Anticancer Agents Med Chem. 2022 Apr 18. DOI: 10.2174/18715206226 66220418141640. Epub ahead of print. PMID: 35440318

[10] Mohanraj V, Chen Y. Nanoparticles—A review. Tropical Journal of Pharmaceutical Research. 2006;**5**(1):561-573

[11] Bazak R et al. Cancer active targeting by nanoparticles: A comprehensive review of literature. Journal of Cancer Research and Clinical Oncology. 2015;**141**(5):769-784

[12] Bhattacharya S. Fabrication of poly(sarcosine), poly (ethylene glycol), and poly (lactic-co-glycolic acid) polymeric nanoparticles for cancer drug delivery. Journal of Drug Delivery Science and Technology. 2021;**61**:102194

[13] Hans ML, Lowman AM. Biodegradable nanoparticles for drug delivery and targeting. Current Opinion in Solid State and Materials Science. 2002;**6**(4):319-327

[14] Golombek SK et al. Tumor targeting via EPR: Strategies to enhance patient responses. Advanced Drug Delivery Review. 2018;**130**:17-38

[15] Khadka P et al. Pharmaceutical particle technologies: An approach to improve drug solubility, dissolution and bioavailability. Asian Journal of Pharmaceutical Sciences. 2014;**9**(6):304-316

[16] Sun T et al. Engineered nanoparticles for drug delivery in cancer therapy. Angewandte Chemie (International ed. in English). 2014;**53**(46):12320-12364

[17] Pérez-Herrero E, Fernández-Medarde AJ. Advanced Targeted Therapies in Cancer: Drug Nanocarriers, the Future of Chemotherapy. European Journal of Pharmaceutics and Biopharmaceutics: Official Journal of Arbeitsgemeinschaft

für Pharmazeutische Verfahrenstechnik e.V. 2015;**93**:52-79

[18] Xie J et al. Therapeutic nanoparticles based on curcumin and bamboo charcoal nanoparticles for chemo-photothermal synergistic treatment of cancer and radioprotection of normal cells. ACS Applied Materials & Interfaces. 2017;**9**(16):14281-14291

[19] Ma Y et al. Polyacrylic acid functionalized Co0. 85Se nanoparticles: An ultrasmall pH-responsive nanocarrier for synergistic photothermal-chemo treatment of cancer. ACS Biomaterials Science & Engineering. 2018;**4**(2):547-557

[20] Hu C et al. Treating cancer stem cells and cancer metastasis using glucose-coated gold nanoparticles. International Journal of Nanomedicine. 2015;**10**:2065

[21] Gordon S, Plüddemann AJF. The mononuclear phagocytic system. Generation of diversity. Frontiers in Immunology. 2019;**10**:1893

[22] Gref R et al. The controlled intravenous delivery of drugs using PEG-coated sterically stabilized nanospheres. Advanced Drug Delivery Reviews. 2012;**64**:316-326

[23] Yapa AS et al. Peptide nanosponges designed for rapid uptake by leukocytes and neural stem cells. RSC Advances. 2018;**8**(29):16052-16060

[24] Ernsting MJ et al. Factors controlling the pharmacokinetics, biodistribution and intratumoral penetration of nanoparticles. Journal of Controlled Release: Official Journal of the Controlled Release Society. 2013;**172**(3):782-794

[25] Anchordoquy TJ, Barenholz Y, Boraschi D, Chorny M, Decuzzi P, Dobrovolskaia MA, et al. ACS Nano. 2017;**11**(1):12-18. DOI: 10.1021/acsnano.6b08244

[26] Maeda H. Polymer therapeutics and the EPR effect. Journal of Drug Targeting. 2017;**25**(9-10):781-785

[27] Maeda H. Toward a full understanding of the EPR effect in primary and metastatic tumors as well as issues related to its heterogeneity. Advanced Drug Delivery Reviews. 2015;**91**:3-6

[28] Walker C, Mojares E, del Río Hernández A. Role of extracellular matrix in development and cancer progression. International Journal of Molecular Sciences. 2018;**19**(10):3028

[29] Dolor A, Szoka FC Jr. Digesting a path forward: the utility of collagenase tumor treatment for improved drug delivery. Molecular Pharmaceutics. 2018;**15**(6):2069-2083

[30] Murphy G, Nagase HJ. Progress in matrix metalloproteinase research. Molecular Aspects of Medicine. 2008;**29**(5):290-308

[31] Wojtowicz-Praga SM, Dickson RB, Hawkins MJ. Matrix metalloproteinase inhibitors. Journal of New Anticancer Agents. 1997;**15**(1):61-75

[32] Wang T-Y et al. Collagen-targeted theranostic nanosponges for delivery of the matrix metalloproteinase 14 inhibitor naphthofluorescein. Chemistry of Materials. 2020;**32**(9):3707-3714

[33] Heldin C-H et al. High interstitial fluid pressure—An obstacle in cancer therapy. Nature Reviews. Cancer. 2004;**4**(10):806-813

[34] Raghunand N, Gillies RJ. pH and drug resistance in tumors. Drug

Resistance Updates: Reviews and Commentaries in Antimicrobial and Anticancer Chemotherapy. 2000;**3**(1):39-47

[35] Vito A, El-Sayes N, Mossman K. Hypoxia-driven immune escape in the tumor microenvironment. Cell. 2020;**9**(4):992

[36] Dai Y et al. Nanoparticle design strategies for enhanced anticancer therapy by exploiting the tumour microenvironment. Chemical Society Reviews. 2017;**46**(12):3830-3852

[37] Caldera F et al. Cyclic nigerosyl-1, 6-nigerose-based nanosponges: An innovative pH and time-controlled nanocarrier for improving cancer treatment. Carbohydrate Polymers. 2018;**194**:111-121

[38] Biswas S, Torchilin VP. Nanopreparations for organelle-specific delivery in cancer. Advanced Drug Delivery Reviews. 2014;**66**:26-41

[39] Nel AE et al. Understanding biophysicochemical interactions at the nano–bio interface. Nature Materials. 2009;**8**(7):543-557

[40] Bannunah AM et al. Mechanisms of nanoparticle internalization and transport across an intestinal epithelial cell model: Effect of size and surface charge. Molecular Pharmaceutics. 2014;**11**(12):4363-4373

[41] Singh P et al. Biofunctionalization of β-cyclodextrin nanosponges using cholesterol. Carbohydrate Polymers. 2018;**190**:23-30

[42] Behzadi S et al. Cellular uptake of nanoparticles: Journey inside the cell. Chemical Society Reviews. 2017;**46**(14):4218-4244

[43] Yan H et al. Engineering cell membrane-based nanotherapeutics to target inflammation. Advanced Science. 2019;**6**(15):1900605

[44] Xue X, Liang X-J. Overcoming drug efflux-based multidrug resistance in cancer with nanotechnology. Chinese Journal of Cancer. 2012;**31**(2):100

[45] Yang X, Liu K. P-gp inhibition-based strategies for modulating pharmacokinetics of anticancer drugs: An update. Current Drug Metabolism. 2016;**17**(8):806-826

[46] Arima H et al. Contribution of P-glycoprotein to the enhancing effects of dimethyl-β-cyclodextrin on oral bioavailability of tacrolimus. Journal of Pharmacology and Experimental Therapeutics. 2001;**297**(2):547-555

[47] Pandey P, Purohit D, Dureja H. Nanosponges–A promising novel drug delivery system. Recent Patents on Nanotechnology. 2018;**12**(3):180-191

[48] Shivani S, Poladi KK. Nanosponges-novel emerging drug delivery system: A review. International Journal of Pharmaceutical Sciences and Research. 2015;**6**(2):529

[49] Ghurghure S, Pathan M, S urwase P. Nanosponges: A novel approach for targeted drug delivery system. International Journal of Chemistry Study. 2018;**2**(6):15-23

[50] Ananya K et al. Recent review on nano sponge. International Journal of Research in Pharmaceutical Sciences. 2020;**11**(1):1085-1096

[51] Swaminathan S, Cavalli R, Trotta F. Cyclodextrin-based nanosponges: A versatile platform for cancer nanotherapeutics development. Wiley Interdisciplinary Reviews:

Nanomedicine and Nanobiotechnology. 2016;**8**(4):579-601

[52] Caldera F et al. Evolution of cyclodextrin nanosponges. International Journal of Pharmaceutics. 2017;**531**(2):470-479

[53] Dhakar NK. Metal and Metal Oxide Nanosponges. Nanosponges: Synthesis and Applications. 2019

[54] Davankov V et al. From a dissolved polystyrene coil to an intramolecularly-hyper-cross-linked "Nanosponge". Macromolecules. 1996;**29**(26):8398-8403

[55] Sherje AP et al. Cyclodextrin-based nanosponges: A critical review. Carbohydrate Polymers. 2017;**173**:37-49

[56] Sadjadi S, Heravi MM, Malmir M. Bio-assisted synthesized Ag (0) nanoparticles immobilized on SBA-15/cyclodextrin nanosponge adduct: Efficient heterogeneous catalyst for the ultrasonic-assisted synthesis of benzopyranopyrimidines. Applied Organometallic Chemistry. 2018;**32**(4):e4286

[57] Thakre A, Gholse Y, Kasliwal R. Nanosponges: A novel approach of drug delivery system. Journal of Medical Pharmaceutical and Allied Sciences. 2016;**78**(92):78

[58] Solunke RS, UDAY RB, Murthy K, Deshmukh MT, RAJKUMAR VS. Formulation and evaluation of gliclazide nanosponges. International Journal of Applied Pharmaceutics. 2019;**11**(6):181-189

[59] Osmani RA et al. Cyclodextrin Nanosponges in Drug Delivery and Nanotherapeutics. In: Dasgupta N, Ranjan S, Lichtfouse E (editors). Environmental Nanotechnology. Environmental Chemistry for a Sustainable World, Springer, Cham. 2018;**14**. DOI:10.1007/978-3-319-76090-2_9

[60] Salunke A, Upmanyu N. Formulation, Development and Evaluation of Budesonide Oral Nano-sponges Using DOE Approach: In Vivo Evidences. Advanced Pharmaceutical Bulletin. 2021 Feb;**11**(2):286-294. DOI:10.34172/apb.2021.041. Epub 2020 Aug 5. PMID: 33880350; PMCID: PMC8046401

[61] Bezawada S, Charanjitha RV, Naveena GV. Nanosponges: A concise review for emerging trends. International Journal of Pharmaceutical Research and Biomedical Analysis. 2014;**3**(1):1-6

[62] Rao MR, Shirsath C. Enhancement of bioavailability of non-nucleoside reverse transcriptase inhibitor using nanosponges. AAPS PharmSciTech. 2017;**18**(5):1728-1738

[63] Jasim IK, Abd Alhammid SN, Abdulrasool AA. Synthesis and evaluation of B-cyclodextrin based nanosponges of 5-fluorouracil by using ultrasound assisted method. Iraqi Journal of Pharmaceutical Sciences. 2020;**29**(2):88-98

[64] Ghosh S, Jagirdar BR. A capping agent dissolution method for the synthesis of metal nanosponges and their catalytic activity towards nitroarene reduction under mild conditions. Dalton Transactions. 2018;**47**(48):17401-17411

[65] Jain A et al. Engineered nanosponges as versatile biodegradable carriers: An insight. Journal of Drug Delivery Science and Technology. 2020;**57**:101643

[66] Tejashri G, Amrita B, Darshana J. Cyclodextrin based nanosponges for pharmaceutical use: A review. Acta Pharmaceutica. 2013;**63**(3):335-358

[67] Allahyari S et al. Cyclodextrin-based nanosponges as promising carriers for

active agents. Expert Opinion on Drug Delivery. 2019;**16**(5):467-479

[68] Osmani AM et al. Nanosponge carriers-an archetype swing in cancer therapy: A comprehensive review. Current Drug Targets. 2017;**18**(1):108-118

[69] Pawar S, Shende P. A comprehensive patent review on β-cyclodextrin cross-linked Nanosponges for multiple applications. Recent Patents on Nanotechnology. 2020;**14**(1):75-89

[70] Krabicová I et al. History of cyclodextrin nanosponges. Polymers. 2020;**12**(5):1122

[71] Bachkar BA et al. Nanosponges: A potential nanocarrier for targeted drug delivery. World Journal of Pharmaceutical Research. 2015;**4**(3): 751-768

[72] Kumar S, Trotta F, Rao R. Encapsulation of babchi oil in cyclodextrin-based nanosponges: Physicochemical characterization, photodegradation, and in vitro cytotoxicity studies. Pharmaceutics. 2018;**10**(4):169

[73] Omar SM, Ibrahim F, Ismail A. Formulation and evaluation of cyclodextrin-based nanosponges of griseofulvin as pediatric oral liquid dosage form for enhancing bioavailability and masking bitter taste. Saudi Pharmaceutical Journal. 2020;**28**(3):349-361

[74] Gangadharappa H, Prasad SMC, Singh RP. Formulation, in vitro and in vivo evaluation of celecoxib nanosponge hydrogels for topical application. Journal of Drug Delivery Science and Technology. 2017;**41**:488-501

[75] Garrido B et al. Carbonate-β-cyclodextrin-based nanosponge as a nanoencapsulation system for piperine: Physicochemical characterization. Journal of Soil Science and Plant Nutrition. 2019;**19**(3):620-630

[76] Rastegar R et al. Evaluation of a novel biocompatible magnetic nanomedicine based on beta-cyclodextrin, loaded doxorubicin-curcumin for overcoming chemoresistance in breast cancer. Artificial Cells, Nanomedicine, and Biotechnology. 2018;**46**(sup. 2):207-216

[77] Gigliotti CL et al. In vitro and in vivo therapeutic evaluation of camptothecin-encapsulated β-cyclodextrin nanosponges in prostate cancer. Journal of Biomedical Nanotechnology. 2016;**12**(1):114-127

[78] Gholibegloo E et al. Folic acid decorated magnetic nanosponge: An efficient nanosystem for targeted curcumin delivery and magnetic resonance imaging. Journal of Colloid and Interface Science. 2019;**556**:128-139

[79] Shringirishi M et al. Fabrication and characterization of nifedipine loaded β-cyclodextrin nanosponges: An in vitro and in vivo evaluation. Journal of Drug Delivery Science and Technology. 2017;**41**:344-350

[80] Penjuri SCB et al. Formulation and evaluation of lansoprazole loaded Nanosponges. Turkish Journal of Pharmaceutical Sciences. 2016;**13**(3):304-310

[81] Moin A et al. Design and formulation of polymeric nanosponge tablets with enhanced solubility for combination therapy. RSC Advances. 2020;**10**(57):34869-34884

[82] Kamble M et al. Formulation optimization and biopharmaceutical evaluation of imatinib mesylate loaded β-cyclodextrin nanosponges.

Pharmaceutical Nanotechnology. 2019;7(5):343-361

[83] Osmani RAM et al. A 3 2 full factorial design for development and characterization of a nanosponge-based intravaginal in situ gelling system for vulvovaginal candidiasis. RSC Advances. 2016;**6**(23):18737-18750

[84] Shah N et al. Development of risedronate sodium-loaded nanosponges by experimental design: Optimization and in vitro characterization. Indian Journal of Pharmaceutical Sciences. 2019;**81**(2):309-316

[85] Pawar S, Shende P. Dual drug delivery of cyclodextrin crosslinked artemether and lumefantrine nanosponges for synergistic action using 23 full factorial designs. Colloids and Surfaces A: Physicochemical and Engineering Aspects. 2020;**602**:125049

[86] Argenziano M et al. In vitro enhanced skin permeation and retention of imiquimod loaded in β-cyclodextrin nanosponge hydrogel. Pharmaceutics. 2019;**11**(3):138

[87] Mady FM, Ibrahim SR. Cyclodextrin-based nanosponge for improvement of solubility and oral bioavailability of Ellagic acid. Pakistan Journal of Pharmaceutical Sciences. 2018 Sep;**31** (5(Supplementary)):2069-2076. PMID: 30393214

[88] Umesh C. Utility of Thiol-Maleimide Click Chemistry for the Synthesis of [2] Rotaxanes Based Novel Polymeric Materials and Protein Conjugates. 2016

[89] Yakavets I et al. Cyclodextrin nanosponge as a temoporfin nanocarrier: Balancing between accumulation and penetration in 3D tumor spheroids. European Journal of Pharmaceutics and Biopharmaceutics. 2020;**154**:33-42

[90] Wang D, Schaaf P. Synthesis and characterization of size controlled bimetallic nanosponges. Physical Sciences Reviews. 2019;**4**(6)163-175

[91] Maity A et al. Catalytic nanosponges of acidic aluminosilicates for plastic degradation and CO 2 to fuel conversion. Nature Communications. 2020;**11**(1):1-12

[92] Rezaei A et al. Improving the solubility and in vitro cytotoxicity (anticancer activity) of ferulic acid by loading it into cyclodextrin nanosponges. International Journal of Nanomedicine. 2019;**14**:4589

[93] Dhakar NK et al. Comparative evaluation of solubility, cytotoxicity and photostability studies of resveratrol and oxyresveratrol loaded nanosponges. Pharmaceutics. 2019;**11**(10):545

[94] Appleton SL et al. Nanosponges as protein delivery systems: Insulin, a case study. International Journal of Pharmaceutics. 2020;**590**:119888

[95] Simionato I et al. Encapsulation of cinnamon oil in cyclodextrin nanosponges and their potential use for antimicrobial food packaging. Food and Chemical Toxicology. 2019;**132**:110647

[96] Wang J et al. Nonviolent self-catabolic DNAzyme nanosponges for smart anticancer drug delivery. ACS Nano. 2019;**13**(5):5852-5863

[97] Argenziano M et al. Improvement in the anti-tumor efficacy of doxorubicin nanosponges in in vitro and in mice bearing breast tumor models. Cancers. 2020;**12**(1):162

[98] Momin MM et al. Extended release delivery of erlotinib glutathione nanosponge for targeting lung cancer.

Artificial Cells, Nanomedicine, and Biotechnology. 2018;**46**(5):1064-1075

[99] Clemente N et al. Paclitaxel-loaded nanosponges inhibit growth and angiogenesis in melanoma cell models. Frontiers in Pharmacology. 2019;**10**:776

[100] Argenziano M et al. Glutathione/pH-responsive nanosponges enhance strigolactone delivery to prostate cancer cells. Oncotarget. 2018;**9**(88):35813

[101] Allahyari S et al. Preparation and characterization of cyclodextrin nanosponges for bortezomib delivery. Expert Opinion on Drug Delivery. 2020;**17**(12):1807-1816

[102] Zhang K et al. DNA nanosponge for adsorption and clearance of intracellular miR-21 and enhanced antitumor chemotherapy. ACS Applied Materials & Interfaces. 2019;**11**(50):46604-46613

[103] Femminò SF, Bessone F, Caldera R, Cavalli F, Trotta P, Pagliaro, et al. Nanosponge-cyclodextrins functionalized with oxygen protects H9C2 cells from hypoxia/reoxygenation injury: Implications from an in vitro model. 2018:54-55

[104] Chen M, Chen M, He J. Cancer cell membrane cloaking nanoparticles for targeted co-delivery of doxorubicin and PD-L1 siRNA. Artificial Cells, Nanomedicine, and Biotechnology. 2019;**47**(1):1635-1641

[105] Li G, Pei M, Liu P. DOX-conjugated CQD-based nanosponges for tumor intracellular pH-triggered DOX release and imaging. Colloids and Surfaces A: Physicochemical and Engineering Aspects. 2020;**603**:125258

[106] Zheng T et al. Gold-nanosponge-based multistimuli-responsive drug vehicles for targeted chemo-photothermal therapy. Advanced Materials. 2016;**28**(37):8218-8226

[107] Su Y-L et al. The penetrated delivery of drug and energy to tumors by lipo-graphene nanosponges for photolytic therapy. ACS Nano. 2016;**10**(10):9420-9433

[108] Hashim DP. Three-dimensional Carbon Nanotube Sponge Materials as Absorbers of Phase Change Materials. USA: WIPO, Editor; 2020

[109] Paliwal H, Parihar A, Prajapati BG. Current state-of-the-art and new trends in self-assembled nanocarriers as drug delivery systems. Frontiers in Nanotechnology. 2022;**4**:836674. DOI: 10.3389/fnano

[110] Bhattacharya S. Methotrexate-loaded polymeric lipid hybrid nanoparticles (PLHNPs): A reliable drug delivery system for the treatment of glioblastoma. Journal of Experimental Nanoscience. 2021;**16**:344-367

Chapter 5

Organogel: A Propitious Carman in Drug Delivery System

Anjali Bedse, Deepa Singh, Shilpa Raut, Kajal Baviskar, Aarti Wable, Prajwal Pagare, Samruddha Wavikar and Samiksha Pagar

Abstract

A gel is a semi-solid formulation having an external solvent phase that is either apolar (organogels) or polar (hydrogels) that is immobilized inside the voids contained in a three-dimensional networked structure. Organogels are bi-continuous systems composed of apolar solvents and gelators. When used at a concentration of around 15%, the gelators form self-assembled fibrous structures that become entangled with one another, resulting in the formation of a three-dimensional networked structure. The resulting three-dimensional networked structure blocks the flow of the external apolar phase. Sterol, sorbitan monostearate, lecithin, and cholesteryl anthraquinone derivatives are examples of gelators. The unique characteristics such as thermo-reversibility, viscoelasticity, and versatility impart a longer shelf-life, prolonged drug release, and patient compliance. These characteristics can easily be adjusted by simple formulation modifications, resulting in highly-structured architectures. Organogels are more likely to be used in various types of delivery systems because of their ability to entrap both hydrophilic and hydrophobic molecules inside their structure. Their combination with other materials allows for tailoring their potential as dosage forms. Organogels have potential applicability in numerous ways; hence this article discusses the various aspects of it.

Keywords: organogels, organogelators, drug delivery, lecithin

1. Introduction

Gels are defined as semisolid, cross-linked systems containing condensed solid particles interpenetrated by a liquid [1]. Gels can be referred to as hydrogels or organogels, which can be distinguished on the basis of polarity comprised by the gel, that is, if the liquid phase in the gel is water then it is referred to as a hydrogel, whereas if the liquid phase in the gel is an apolar solvent, then it is referred as an organogel. Organogels are the carriers used for delivering the medicament at its desired site [2]. Organogels are formed by gelators, which are foundational building blocks. Gelators are often certain low-molecular-mass substances (e.g., sorbitan derivatives, lecithin, fatty acid derivatives, bis-urea compounds) [3–5]. The gelators help in the formation of a 3D structure of a mesh network due to the entanglement of self-assembled fibrous structures, which are formed due to some physical or chemical interactions of gelators when used in the concentration of <15% (approx.) [6, 7]. Gelators are hence responsible for immobilizing the apolar solvent phase. The gels formed by the physical interactions are termed physical gels (held by physical forces such as Van der Waals and hydrogen bonds) whereas the gels formed by chemical bonding are termed chemical gels (held by covalent bonds) [7]. The gelators elevate the surface tension which predominantly prevents the flow of the solvent phase. Gelators immobilize organic solvents by the establishment of non-covalent intermolecular interactions forces (H-bonds, electrostatic interactions, metal coordination, p–p stacking, and London dispersion forces), resulting in the formation of various entangled structures like wrinkles, lamellar, and fibers [8–11]. The thermo-reversible property, non-irritating nature, and biocompatibility of the organogels have generated much interest in their potential application as a drug delivery system. Wide formulations can be developed for the administration of drugs via various routes using organogels as they can incorporate hydrophilic and hydrophobic bioactive agents within their gel structure. The rate-limiting step in the bioavailability of drugs from organogels is its characteristic features, that is, high permeability, and low aqueous solubility, which affect the rate of drug release from drug delivery systems. They have no confined application as they can be used for topical application or for the release of drugs into systemic circulation by cutaneous delivery and percutaneous absorption [7, 12].

2. Types of organogel

2.1 Lecithin organogels (LOs)

Since LOs have the desirable physicochemical characteristics ideal for topical formulations, these are employed most frequently for topical application. These are useful for the delivery of a wide variety of hydrophilic as well as lipophilic drugs through the skin. Lecithin is a constituent of natural origin which can be isolated from various animal and plant sources (except egg yolk) and hence biocompatible, safe and stable [7, 13, 14]. It is a potential vehicle for a number of bioactive agents. Lecithin is chemically a phosphatidylcholine, a constituent of the class phospholipids. It has been observed that lecithin is unable to form a gel if its phosphatidyl content is less than 95% [7, 15]. The concept of designing organogels with lecithin was first mentioned by Luisi and Scartazzini in the year 1988 [16]. Lecithin can only produce gelation if it is used in its pure form (e.g., the hydrogenated form of soya-lecithin failed to induce gelation). The unsaturated fatty acids present in naturally occurring lecithin are hence important [15].

2.2 Pluronic lecithin organogels (PLOs)

High-purity lecithin is costly and difficult to procure in significant quantities. Due to the convenience of synthetic polymers such as pluronics, which serve as co-surfactant and stabilizers, they have been widely studied in combination with lecithin to formulate lecithin micro-emulsion-based organogels [17]. It was prepared in 1990 in the US by a compounding pharmacist to use as a topical carrier system [15]. The primary benefit of employing PLs in organogels is their capacity to self-assemble into micelles at approximate physiological temperatures [11]. Pluronic F-127 is a copolymer which causes gelation when used in a concentration of 15–30% w/v [18]. It is formed by adding the Pluronic F-127 to the LOs. It is majorly used for transdermal as well as topical drug delivery systems and also for oral and mucosal drug delivery systems to some extent [15]. It forms a non-transparent yellow gel [19]. After topical administration, PLOs rupture the lipid layer of the stratum corneum and deliver the drug into the systemic circulation with minimal irritation to the skin [7, 18]. Additionally, in order to have a synergistic effect, it has also been demonstrated to be a useful transporter for combinations of drugs [20]. It works best when combined with medications whose molecular weight is less than 500 Da [21].

2.3 Limonene GP1/PG organogels

Limonene is a terpenoid with magnificent penetration power and is used in transdermal drug delivery systems as it can enhance the bioavailability of drugs [22]. This organogel is prepared by mixing a suitable amount of GP1 (dibutyllauroylbutamide) amino acid type of organogelator with limonene and PG (propylene glycol), followed by its incubation at 120°C. After cooling down to an appropriate temperature, it forms a gel that appears white in color. It has been observed that the co-existence of limonene with GP1 and PG influences its rheological behavior to some extent, whereas their chemical characteristics are not significantly affected [7, 15, 19, 23]. The GP1/PG organogels tend to have increased gel moduli due to the incorporation of limonene, which gives an indication of increased gel physical stability [24]. Other terpenoids such as cineole and linalool, have also been successfully mixed with GP1 and PG to obtain an effective organogel with improved penetration power [18].

2.4 Micro-emulsion-based organogels (MBG) stabilized by gelatin

Micro-emulsions offer good bioavailability of drugs when introduced via topical or systemic routes of the drug delivery systems. Micro-emulsions are known to deliver a greater amount of drug than other gel systems [15]. The micro-emulsion system can undergo gelation when gelatin is dissolved in the water microphase, and the resultant gel will consist of more than 80% hydrocarbon solvent [25]. The basic mechanism involved in the formation of MBG is that a solution of gelatin in water is added to the parent micro-emulsion after it has been incubated at 50°C in the incubation chamber. In order to obtain an optically transparent single-phase gel, the resulting liquid is forcefully mixed and then allowed to cool to ambient temperature [26]. Gelatin is a protein that has the ability to form gels. It can undergo gelation when its concentrated solution is heated beyond 45°C and is then cooled down below 35°C and increases thermostability. When gelatin is added to w/o micro-emulsions, a transparent gel of the complete micellar solution is obtained [7, 15, 19, 27, 28].

2.5 Sorbitan organogels derived from fatty acids

Sorbitan monopalmitate (span 40) and Sorbitan monostearate (span 60) are the gelators of this class. They are non-ionic, hydrophobic in nature, and possess surfactant properties. They form a solid-fiber matrix when heated with the apolar solvent and then cooled down to a relatively lower temperature. A gel of toroidal reverse micelle is formed due to a drop in the temperature, which is followed by self-assembly leading to its transformation into rod-shaped tubules. The gel so obtained is white, opaque, semisolid, and thermostable at room temperature. These organogels are used as vehicles for hydrophilic vaccines [29–31].

2.6 Polyethylene organogels

Low molecular-weight polyethylene is solubilized in mineral oil at a high temperature of more than 130°C, yielding a colorless organogel. This causes intermolecular interaction within the polyethylene, which leads to the precipitation of its molecules, which forms a solid-fiber matrix to form a gel [16]. They are generally used as a base for ointment preparations [19]. A study conducted in the 1950s concluded that the patches of polyethylene organogel were found to be non-irritating along with low sensitizing properties [15].

2.7 Eudragit organogels

Eudragit organogels are formed by the mixture of polyhydric alcohols (propylene glycol and glycerol), a high concentration (30–40%) of Eudragit (L or S), and liquid PEG. To prepare a formulated Eudragit organogel, the drug is first dissolved in the PEG, and this solution is then added to the Eudragit powder. This mixture is further triturated with the help of a mortar and pestle for approximately 1 minute. The concentration of Eudragit and the amount of drug are found to directly influence the consistency of the gel. The gel viscosity is enhanced with a high concentration of Eudragit, whereas it decreases with an increasing amount of the drug. In low concentrations of drugs, the gel has high rigidity as well as stability [7, 15].

2.8 Supramolecular organogels

These organogels are made of gelators of low molecular mass. The molecules of different gelators of this class differ immensely in their structural characteristics. Hence, they have offered a scope of interest to develop different gels with technological application. For example, having sensitivity toward external stimuli like light. Remarkable thermoreversibility and mechanical capabilities are displayed by supramolecular organogel systems with controlled self-assembled structures. These organogels can offer controlled drug delivery. They can be used as carriers for multiple purposes [15, 32].

2.9 L-alanine-derived organogels

LAM (N-lauroyl-L-alanine methylester) undergoes gelation with organic solvents such as triglycerides and soya-bean oil. It is not as extensively used as other organogels. At room temperature, it remains in a gel state [7, 15, 18]. In a biphasic mixture of water and apolar solvent, a fatty acid derivative of L-alanine aids the gelling of the solvent-specific portion of the mixture without gelling the aqueous portion [33]. This characteristic makes it considerably more appealing to use in organogel. It can be used as an implant for sustained release system. Currently, it is used as a vehicle for the drugs like leuprolide, rivastigmine [7, 18].

3. Importance of organogels

For the conveyance of medications in the body/target site, numerous procedures and frameworks have been analyzed. Out of the effective applications accessible, organogels are getting greater fame on account of the simplicity of utilization, better ingestion through the skin layers, etc. Amongst the existing dosage forms, organogels are the easiest to prepare and have also been proven to be cost-effective [7, 34, 35]. They offer a better stability profile than that of other gels. The characteristic features of organogels not only make it easier for the manufacturer to process but also provide an easy handling and utilization method for the consumers, hence making it of commercial importance. The organogels can deliver the drugs more effectively than other dosage forms. This has been validated through a study which was conducted by I.M. Shaikh et al., where it was observed that the penetration efficiency of organogel (LO) was greater than that of hydrogels when applied over skin [35, 36]. As it offers a controlled drug delivery system, many chronic diseases could be cured if the organogels are loaded with appropriate drugs and then implanted at the target site. This characteristic also eliminates the obligation of frequent dosing. They have an extended application as they lend opportunities to incorporate various constituents having wide-ranging characteristics. Organogels can be used as an alternative to UV-treatment methods. Hence, it will eliminate the chances of cancer caused by exposure to UV rays [37, 38]. Organogel can reduce/control the dissemination rate of medication, hence making it liable for designing an appropriate formulation for an appropriate purpose to deliver the drug as required. As it comprises both hydrophilic and lipophilic parts, both lipophilic and hydrophilic bioactive agents could be consolidated within it [15, 38]. Therefore, wide-ranging drugs could be incorporated into them.

4. Advantages of organogels

It is an easy formulation to prepare and has a longer life span. Bioactive agents of distinct characteristics can be incorporated [37, 38]. Their physical form remains unaffected by the factor of time owing to structural cohesion. It is cost-effective as it requires a lower number of components [37–39]. They have simple handling and usage requirements. It also provides improved patient compliance [34]. It has various applications for topical delivery systems. It has thermal stability [38]. A few chemical modifications can lead to the release of drugs in the desired manner and at the desired place [34]. It bypasses first-pass metabolism, ensuring that medicines have the highest possible bioavailability. They are relatively safe as bio-compatible constituents are used. Hence, it can be used to deliver various drugs. It is non-invasive and is better tolerated by the patients. It is a thermodynamically stable system. As it can be used for an extended period of time, the need for dosing is less frequent. It has both hydrophobic and hydrophilic units. Therefore, bioactive agents of either nature can be incorporated into it. There is no risk of microbial contamination as they are insensitive to moisture [34, 38].

5. Limitations

It accounts for low thermostability. It has a greasy texture [2]. For the drugs that are intended to be penetrated through the skin, they must possess an appropriate partition coefficient. It holds good chances for the occurrence of swelling (uptake of liquid resulting in an increase in its volume) or syneresis (natural shrinkage if allowed to be at rest for a period of time) [15, 40]. Organogels intended for topical application might irritate the local skin. Topical organogels cannot comprise bioactive agents with molecular weights of more than 500 Dalton, since skin can be permeated by drugs with molecular weights under 500 Dalton [18]. The purity of the constituents present is important, or else there might be no gel formation. Few organogelators are not available on a large scale, hence causing expense elevation for formulation, for example, lecithin organogelator. The purity of the constituents present is important, or else there might be no gel formation. Precise control of process variables (pH, temperature, etc.) is mandatory. Skin permeation enhancers and non-polar solvents are added in order to achieve deep penetration through skin, which may produce toxicity. Because of the gelator and the necessary solvent used, it is difficult to determine whether the gelation process will be successful [41].

6. Properties of organogel

A few characteristic attributes that organogels possess include non-invasiveness, non-toxicity, etc. But its substantial physicochemical properties, which frame it as a significant and essential system, are as follows.

6.1 Viscoelasticity

The term "viscoelasticity" is related to the materials that possess the two properties, that is, viscosity and elasticity. The viscoelastic property of organogels has also been authenticated by stress relaxation studies [6, 42]. They act as solids at lower shear stress (elasticity) and as a flowing fluid at escalated shear stress [15, 38]. At low shear rates, there is no pressure acting over them; hence they behave like solids with an intact structure, but at higher shear stress, as the pressure increases, the 3D-mesh network within the structure starts rupturing, permitting it to flow. It is observed that the organogels appear to follow the Maxwell model of viscoelasticity. It is observed that they retain plastic-flow behavior. "Organogels" are similar to other gel systems; the gelling agent creates an ongoing, three-dimensional network in the solvent, obstructing the flow of liquid. The rheological behavior of the gelator solution and its interaction with the solvent can greatly influence the flow property of the organogels [6, 15].

6.2 Thermostability

The nature of the organogels makes them innately thermostable. The capability of the gelators to undergo self-assembly under suitable conditions to produce organogels may be responsible for the stability of the organogels. The overall free energy of the system decreases when the gelators undergo self-assembly, yielding a low-energy thermostable organogel. At elevated temperatures, the molecules within the organogels acquire some kinetic energy to reduce any loss in their structure, and low temperatures, they resume their original structure. This innate property of the organogel is responsible for its longer shelf-life, thereby making it ideal for the delivery of bioactive agents [15, 16, 19].

6.3 Thermoreversibility

The matrix structure of the organogel is distorted when it is heated at a temperature that is extended from its critical temperature and hence it starts flowing. This added thermal energy causes interaction amongst the molecules of the organogel, causing disruption in the structure. But as the temperature decelerates, the interaction of the molecules also retards, which results in the reverting back of the organogel to its original configuration. This whole phenomenon is called thermoreversibility property of the organogels. For example, PLOs, when heated above 25°C (critical temperature), lost solid-matrix configuration, and after cooling, and returned to a stable configuration. The fluid matrix systems (Fluid matrix organogels) are thermoreversible [7, 16].

6.4 Non-birefringence

Birefringence is the optical property of a material that allows propagation of light when polarized light passes through it. The organogels are non-birefringent, that is, they do not allow the propagation of light when polarized light passes through their matrix. As a result, when organogels are observed under polarized light, these appear as dark matrix. This can be attributed to the isotropic property of the organogels [16, 19, 29, 43].

6.5 Optical clarity

The transparency or opacity of the organogels will depend on the chemical makeup they possess. For example, sorbitan monostearate organogels and PLOs are opaque, whereas the lecithin organogels are transparent in nature [30, 44].

6.6 Chirality effect

It has been observed that the stability and growth of the solid-fiber networks are both impacted by the presence of chirality in LMW (Low-Molecular Weight) gelators. Additionally, the thermoreversibility of the gels produced as a result of the self-assembled solid-fiber network is related to chirality. A competent solid-fiber gelator has been shown to be generally effective in possessing a chiral center, but fluid-fiber gels are unaffected by chirality. The gelators inclusive of chiral centers aid in the production of a tight molecular packing, hence impart kinetic and thermodynamic stability to organogels. The Crown ether phthalocyanine organogel is a good chiral organogel example [7, 45].

6.7 Biocompatibility

Previously, the organogels were formulated by using several non-biocompatible components, which resulted in non-biocompatible organogels. Currently, research on organogels involving different biocompatible constituents such as vegetable oil and cocoa butter has increased their potential for extended use in biomedical field [15, 19, 38, 40].

7. Organogelators

Organogelators are the gelling agents that have the capability to transform a preparation into a semisolid mass, that is, gel. They are used to impart the desired consistency in organogels. Hence, they are an integral component in the formulation of organogels. The solubility of the organogelator in the solvent generates a few forces, which is the reason for the stability of the thermodynamic and kinetic characteristics of the gel [7]. Organogelators have the property of changing their physical state depending upon the temperature. They remain as a solid matrix at room temperature but transform into liquid at relatively lower temperatures. The structure of organogels mainly depends upon the constructing ability of the organogelator [9]. The degree of cooperative self-assembly in an organogel is also regulated by the gelator structure and solubility [46]. The most manageable type of organogelators are n-alkanes and are useful in gelling the other proportionally short-chained alkanes [2]. It precipitates out as fibers form a 3D-structure. It is mainly responsible for the design/structure of organogels. They produce bond formation within the molecules of organogels, leading to their interaction and bonding amongst each other and an increase in the thickness of the preparation. Depending upon the type of bond they form, organogelators can be regarded as-hydrogen bond forming organogelators, viz., amino acids, amides, carbohydrates, etc., or as non-hydrogen bond forming organogelators, viz., anthraquinone, steroidal moieties, anthracene, etc. [9, 19, 38]. The ongoing research on organogelators has formed a branch for other novel types of gelators, including sugar-based organogelators and green organogelators, etc. [47, 48]. These new types of gelators each have their own concepts that should be studied comprehensively for a better understanding of the widespread availability of organogelators from a variety of sources.

7.1 Types of organogelators

7.1.1 Aryl cyclohexanol derivatives

These are 4-Tertiary Butyl-1-aryl cyclohexanols derivatives. Their characteristic features, which they impart in the gel, may differ depending upon the nature of the apolar solvent involved in the organogel. They possess low solubility in apolar solvents and hence they might appear as a turbid or transparent preparation, depending on the nature of apolar solvent involved. Their physical state is solid at room temperature. They can produce gelation only if the phenyl group in their structure lies in the axial configuration. The derivatives possessing phenyl groups in the equatorial configuration are unable to form the gel. They help in obtaining the organogels with the desired property of thermo-reversibility. A few common examples of this class are CCl4, benzene, cyclohexane, etc.

7.1.2 Polymer organogels

These are long chain-containing gelling agents. These are the gelators that possess a high capability of inducing gelation. They have a molecular size of more than 2 kilo Dalton. They can impart gel formation even if used in very low concentrations. They can appear in different shapes (straight, branched, etc.). Their efficiency of imparting gelation can be modified if their chemical structure is somewhat altered. They can be further divided into physical or chemical organogelators. If they form chemical bonds within the network of organogel, then they are regarded as physical organogelators which result in a cross-linked network, and if they form non-covalent bonds, then they are regarded as chemical organogelators which result in an entangled chain-linked network. The transition temperature for the transformation of the gel state to a sol state is also very low. They have relatively higher gel-strength than other LMOGs. They mostly include L-lysine derivatives and the other conventional examples are polyethylene, polycarbonate, polymethylmethacrylate, polyester, etc. [18, 19, 34, 38, 40].

7.1.3 Gemini organogelator

"Gemini" means "twins". This word has been derived from Latin language. The first Gemini organogelator of L-lysine was synthesized by Suzuki et al. [49]. It had two chains of L-lysine of different chain lengths, linked together by an amide bond. This chain length is inversely proportional to the gelation ability of the gelator. They possess good gelation properties. They have a high ability to immobilize various kinds of apolar solvents. A good example of this class is Bis (N-lauroyl-L-lysine ethyl ester) oxylamide which can immobilize solvents like ketones, alcohols, etc. [9, 18, 19, 38].

7.1.4 Boc-Ala(1)-Aib(2)-β-Ala(3)-OMe organogelators

It is a synthetic tripeptide gelator of synthetic origin. It is capable of undergoing self-CB (1, 2-dichlorobenzene), 1-chlorobenzene, etc.

7.1.5 Low-molecular-weight organogelators (LMWOs)

These are the gelling agents that possess a small molecular weight (≤3000 Dalton) [9, 50]. Assembly which is the contributor of its gel-formation ability. They form thermoreversible and transparent gels. The apolar solvents, to which they can immobilize include benzene. These are most widely used organogelators. They contain a high capability of immobilizing the aqueous phase, even if used in small concentrations (<2%). The length of the alkyl chain in LMWO directly influences its gelling ability [51]. They mostly form solid-fiber matrices or can form fluid-fiber matrices based on the intermolecular interaction they perform. A solid-fiber matrix can be obtained if the organogelator is cooled down beyond the solubility range of the gelator, which is then followed by a rapid, incomplete precipitation, in the organic solvent, which leads to physical intermolecular interactions. For forming a fluid matrix, a polar solvent should be added to the solution of surfactant, leading to the re-arrangement of molecules to form a clump, hence immobilizing the aqueous phase. This also results in a difference in the kinetic-stability between both the matrices, which can be used as a distinguishing factor. Solid-fiber matrix offers an enhanced mechanical property compared to that of fluid-fiber matrix. This is because a solid-fiber matrix contains a highly arranged molecular structure compared to a fluid-fiber matrix. LMOGs have been further categorized into steroidal organogelators, ALS organogelators, etc., depending on the chemical backbone they possess [7, 19, 34, 38, 52].

8. Mechanism of organogelation

Organogelation is generally induced by the incorporation of a polar solvent into the organogel. If lecithin is present in it, then, it forms reverse spherical micelles at a ~ 0.01 mM concentration. This is induced by the addition of a small quantity of polar additives which bind to the hydrophilic head of the lecithin. This creates linear networks. If the amount of polar additive is further increased, then it leads to the formation of long tubular flexible micelles. After overlapping with each other sufficiently, they entangle themselves and build up a transient 3D network (**Figure 1**).

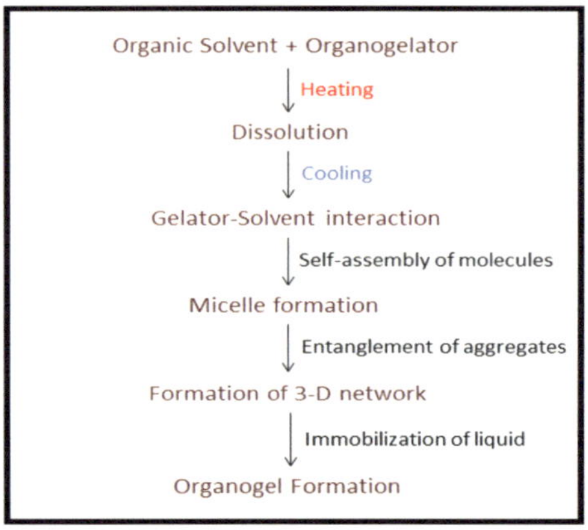

Figure 1.
Mechanism of Organogelation.

In the case of PLOs, the mechanism of gelling and the structural network may be related to the synergistic contribution of both phospholipids and polymeric co-surfactant molecules in their respective hydrated states. In this case, solvent molecules and lecithin phosphate groups can be arranged in such a way that a hydrogen-bonded network will be formed [15, 34, 52].

9. Mechanism of gel permeation into skin

Human skin is made up of different types of tissue layers. The outermost layer, Stratum corneum is the rate limiting barrier for the permeation of gel into the skin [35]. It has been observed that lipid based formulations enhance penetration through the skin; however, they modify the hydration state of the skin, causing dermatitis. Aqueous formulations maintain the skin intact and bioactive, but have less penetration [18]. In the case of Pluronic Lecithin organogels, penetration and permeation are enhanced due to lecithin, which alters the skin structure and transiently opens the skin pores. It is believed that this happens due to the interaction between the lecithin's phospholipid and skin lipids. Hence, there occurs the formation of a cylindrical network which results in an increase in the area of the lecithin polar region, and non-polar solvent acts as a penetration enhancer and then penetration occurs by forming a thin film on the skin surface (**Figure 2**) [16, 18, 35].

10. Method for preparation of organogels

At 60°C, the oil-surfactant mixture is heated to produce a transparent solution that, when cooled, transforms into organogels. Lecithin solutions are made by first dissolving lecithin in organic solvents using a magnetic stirrer, according to the phase diagrams that have been constructed. Organogels are created by adding water with the use of a micropipette syringe. Heat may be used occasionally to completely dissolve drugs. Lecithin and an organic solvent are combined to create the oil phase, which is then let to stand overnight to guarantee full breakdown. When preparing the aqueous (polar) phase, pluronic is added to ice-cold water and stirred to ensure

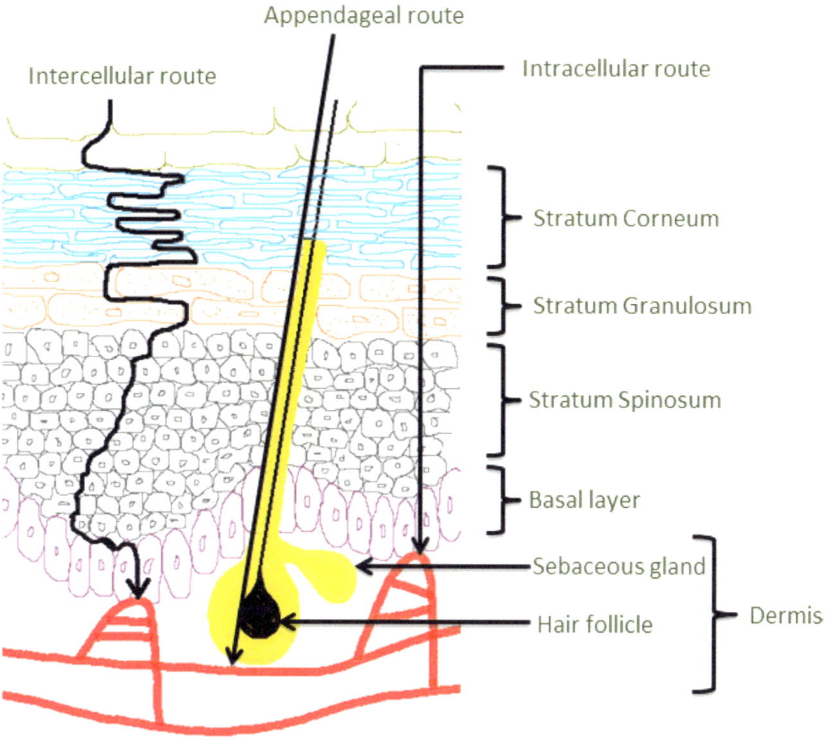

Figure 2.
Pathways for permeation of organogel into skin.

thorough dissolve. The produced PLO is blended with the Pluronic's aqueous phase using a high-shear mixing technique by a magnetic stirrer. Fatty-acid gelators can also be used to create organogels by first dissolving them at a higher temperature in a water-in-oil emulsion, then lowering the temperature. The solubility of the gelator decreases as a result of the drop in temperature, which leads to precipitation and self-assembly of the gelators into a network of tubules that become entangled to create a gelled structure [2, 19].

10.1 Fluid-filled fiber method

It is a well-known technique for making organogels, where in reverse micelles are produced by dissolving surfactants and co-surfactants in an apolar solvent. Reverse micelles are then transformed to tubular reverse micelles after the addition of water. The elongated reverse micelle becomes entangled to create a 3-dimensional network, which immobilizes apolar solvent [53].

10.2 Solid fiber method

In the Solid fiber method, an apolar solvent and solid organogelator are heated together at an apolar solution of the solid organogelator is produced. Then cool it at room temperature, the organogelator precipitates out as fibers that interact physically with one another to form a three-dimensional network structure that immobilizes apolar solvent [15, 38].

Types	Administration Route	Study carried out	Model Drugs	Reference
Sorbitan monostearate	Nasal Oral Subcutaneous & intramuscular	In vitro release In vivo efficacy	Propranolol Cyclosporin A	[55] [56]
Lecithin	Transdermal	Clinical studies Skin permeation and effectiveness in vivo Skin permeation in vitro Skin release in vitro	Metoprolol Aceclofenac Indomethacin Diclofenac Bioactive agents	[57] [13, 58, 59]
Eudragit organogels	Rectal Buccal	In vivo efficacy	Salicylic acid BSA	[44, 60]

Table 1.
Formulations of organogels used in drug delivery.

10.3 Hydration method

In this technique the inorganic chemical is directly hydrated to form the dispersed phase of the dispersion, which is then used to create gel. Other substances such as propylene glycol, propyl gallate, and hydroxypropyl cellulose may be employed in addition to water as a carrier to improve gel formation [53].

10.4 Novel methods

Conventional methods of preparing organogels usually require longer heating times and neutralizing agents. Evren et al. prepared organogels employing a new technique, high-speed homogenization which was followed by microwave heating. Evren et al. prepared Triclosan organogel employing Carbopol 974 NF in PEG 400. Carbopol in varying concentrations (2–4%) was dispersed in PEG 400. The resulting dispersion was homogenized at 24,000 rpm.. The dispersion was heated using two methods. The first involved heating at 80°C, stirring mechanically at 200 rpm. In the second method, the dispersion was subjected to micro-irradiation (1200 W/1 h) for 2 min. The results demonstrated that microwave heating was suitable for preparing carbopol organogels. Owing to significant reduction in time and energy, the method holds good promise for industrial applicability [54] (**Table 1**).

11. Factors affecting organogels

11.1 pH

A pH change stimulates the reversible transition of an organogel from a gel state to a sol state [61]. Hence, pH can influence the physical state of gels.

11.2 Temperature

Organogels are often less stable with increasing temperatures, causing disruption of the 3D mesh-network structure. Temperature also affects viscosity. As the temperature increases, the viscosity decreases [4]. Hence, the temperature range during their storage should be closely controlled [5, 18, 19].

11.3 Organogelator

The type of organogelator used for the preparation has the capability to influence the mechanical and rheological properties of the organogel [40].

11.4 Adjuvants

a. Surfactants: Characteristics of gel can be varied depending upon the surfactant.

b. Salts: The addition of salt to the organogel may result in salting-out (formation of more secondary bonds amongst the molecules) [15, 38].

c. Organic solvent: The structure of an organogel depends upon the nature of the solvent (polar/non-polar).

d. Organogelator: The rate of drug release from the organogel is affected by/depends upon the concentration of the gelator used [62].

e. Skin permeation enhancers: These chemical entities might also possess additional characteristics, which may interact and alter the properties of the organogel.

Terpenes operate as chemical penetration enhancers and also act as rheology modifiers, which may result in any alteration in the flow property and deformation characteristics of an organogel [63].

11.5 Moisture

Organogels swell when exposed to moisture as they absorb water molecules from it This may aid in the instability of the organogels [38].

11.6 Purity

The constituents used in an organogel should be in its pure form. Any impurity in the components may lead to instability in the network of the matrix, for example, lecithin is unable to induce gelation if not used in its pure form [2, 40].

12. Application of organogels

12.1 Pharmaceutical industry

a. Topical drug delivery system.

The skin, being the largest tissue in the body, provides good bioavailability of drugs, as the drugs meant to enter the systemic circulation via permeation through the skin bypass the first-pass metabolism. Pluronic lecithin organogels (PLOs) contain isopropyl myristate/isopropyl palmitate as an apolar organic solvent used as a vector for the release of NSAIDs (ketoprofen, flurbiprofen, diclofenac sodium), used as an analgesic. Reverse micellar MBGs possess soya-lecithin/iso-octane/water as a solvent phase for the delivery of propranolol. Organogels can be regarded as potential matrices for the controlled release of topical antimicrobials. Organogels loaded with Piroxicam are used for the treatment of rheumatoid arthritis. In-situ forming organogel of L-alanine injectable can be used for the release of labile macromolecular drugs. Various studies on formulation of transdermal organogels, such as development of PLO with mometasone furoate for psoriasis and fluconazole-loaded organogels based on olive oil for fungal infections, have exhibited positive results [9, 42, 64].

b. Oral and trans-mucosal drug delivery system.

The drugs can be delivered through oral cavity with the help of implantation of bio-adhesive organogels, that is, the drugs will be administered as implants. The drug can be dissolved within the organic solvent and then mixed with the muco-adhesive polymer. An organogel of 12-HSA-soyabean oil was used for the delivery of ibuprofen [15]. An in-vivo study conducted in rats depicted that the organogels can be employed as a vector for controlled release of lipophilic drugs [38]. Sorbitan monoleate based organogel, incorporated with cyclosporine A is given orally. An oral organogel can be prepared by incorporating an NSAID (ibuprofen) to achieve desired therapeutic results [65].

c. Parenteral drug delivery system.

Parenteral routes are the preferential choice for the administration of drugs, as it avoids first-pass metabolism, provides quicker onset of action, etc. An in-situ forming organogel prepared for sustain delivery of leuprolide (used in prostate cancer) from the L-alanine derivatives in safflower oil and was injected by SC route. It was observed that the gel degraded slowly for drug release over a span of 14–25 days [7, 15]. Sorbitan monostearate organogel preparation have been developed and given by SC and IM route for the release of propranolol/ cyclosporine A/ BSA and HA [7]. A study depicted that, safflower oil-based N-methyl pyrrolidone (NMP) injections were introduced into rats subcutaneously, which was well-tolerated by the surrounding tissues over a period of 8 weeks [66]. The injection of an in-situ organogel forming implant based on SAM (N-stearoyl-L-alanine methyl ester) demonstrated significant promise for safe and suitable delivery method for therapeutic medications that require regulated release [67]. A successful evaluation was conducted for the purpose of using parenteral organogel in schizophrenia therapy [68]. The micro-emulsion based organogels and niosomes containing organogels have been formulated for delivery of vaccines. After administration of these gels via intramuscular route, a depot effect was observed (**Table 2**) [15].

d. Ophthalmic drug delivery system.

Ophthalmic solutions are generally used for administering drugs in the eye, but due to its consistency, frequent dosing is required as the drug may not be properly

Parameters	Description
Gelation Studies	A straightforward visual test to establish whether gelation has been established and includes: inverting the reaction vessel, pouring with organogel; if the sample does not flow, gelation has occurred [40]
Rheological Behavior	An indication of the structural organization of the organogel is obtained by its rheological behavior. The viscosity the usually determined with the help of a Brookfield viscometer [69]
Structural features	Utilizing NMR spectroscopy, the molecular design of organogels has been evaluated, and FTIR spectroscopy has demonstrated hydrogen bonding. Optical microscopy, freeze fracture electron microscopy, transmission electron microscopy and X-ray diffraction have been used to learn about the molecular packing within the organogel network [29, 38]
Phase transition Temperature	It is the determination of the temperature at which the organogel transforms from gel state to sol state. It provides details on the types of the microstructures that make up the cross-linked gelling network. The presence of uniform microstructures within the gel is indicated by a restricted PTT range (3–5°C). Hot stage microscopy (HST) and high sensitivity DCS are employed to determine it. Basically, the organogels are placed in glass tubes which are subjected to incrementing temperature. The transition is analyzed by inverting the tubes and this temperature is then noted [59]
pH	A digital pH meter is used to assess the pH of the formulation. A suitable amount of organogel is dissolved in a solvent. The pH meter electrode is submerged in this mixture, which then display the value of pH [42]
Water Content	Evaporation of water can cause viscosity to drop, which can impair the stability of the gel. The use of NIR spectroscopy (NIR, 1800–2200) to measure water content [59]
Stability study	The stability of organogels can be determined at different temperature and relative humidity conditions as per ICH guidelines. 25°C ± 2°C at 75 ± 5% RH 40°C ± 2°C at 75 ± 5% RH
In vitro studies	Through a dialysis membrane, the formulation is subjected to in vitro diffusion. A Franz diffusion cell can be employed to determine the drug release [2]
In vivo studies	Various animals, such as rats, are employed as models for several evaluation such as skin irritation tests and compatibility tests
Physical examination	It is a preliminary assessment in which, the prepared organogel is evaluated for its color, texture, appearance, odor, etc. [29]

Table 2.
Evaluation of organogels.

absorbed in the target site. Hence thicker preparations like gels are desired to increase the contact time to facilitate the maximum absorption of drugs from the formulation. Methazolamide is incorporated into carbomer and poloxamer gels for the treatment of glaucoma which was ineffective when formulated as ophthalmic solution [38]. Organogelators are employed with drugs such as Eudragit L and S for ophthalmic preparation for sustained delivery [50].

12.2 Food industry

Organogels are primarily employed in the food industry owing to their ability to reduce oil mobility in food items, particularly those containing multiple ingredients. Organogels can be used as replacer for Trans and saturated fat in processed foods to install a specific texture. Wax-based organogels provide good oxidative stability, and also influence the firmness and spreadability and thus can be used in spreadable food product [18, 64, 70].

12.3 Cosmetics industry

Low molecular weight organogelators (LMOGs) such as DBS and 12-HSA are used for preparation of lipsticks [71]. 12-HSA organogelator is used in sunscreens to block UVB rays [41]. It is possible to improve the properties of organogels developed for cosmetic applications by using organic solvents like Amazonian oils, which already possess moisturizing and nourishing effects [72]. Various dermatological cosmetics such as lip-gels, skin, and hair protectants can be prepared in the form of organogels [18, 38]. Other cosmetic preparations such as shampoo, dentifrices, and perfumes are prepared in the form of organogels [15].

13. Conclusion

Organogels are a visco-elastic substance primarily made by gelling the organic solvent with a bioactive agent. It has captivated a section of curiosity to explore all the aspects of their application, as these can potentially eliminate or replace many components, techniques as well as limitations being faced normally for different types of formulations, due to unique properties. The organogels have a huge area for application, although possess few drawbacks and limitations. Though these can be administered to the body via various drug delivery routes, the major site is topical route considering ease of application and many more reasons. A stable organogel designed with all the bio-compatible components might attract the commercial market in future as they can potentially become the preferential choice of formulators and consumers.

Acronyms and abbreviations

LOs	lecithin organogels
PLs	pluronics
PLOs	pluronic lecithin organogels
GP1	dibutyllauroylbutamide
PG	propylene glycol
MBG	micro-emulsion based organogels
w/o	water in oil
span 40	sorbitan monopalmitate
span 60	sorbitan stearate

PEG	poly ethylene glycol
LAM	N-lauroyl-L-alanine methylester
CCl_4	carbon tetrachloride
LMWO	low-molecular-weight organogelators
3D	3 dimensional
NSAIDs	non-steroidal anti-inflammatory drugs
HST	hot stage microscopy
PTT	phase transition temperature
NIR	near infra-red
NMP	N-methyl pyrrolidone
SC	subcutaneous
IM	intramuscular
SAM	N-stearoyl-L-alanine methyl ester
BSA	bovine serum albumin
HA	hemagglutinin

Author details

Anjali Bedse*, Deepa Singh, Shilpa Raut, Kajal Baviskar, Aarti Wable, Prajwal Pagare, Samruddha Wavikar and Samiksha Pagar
Department of Pharmaceutics, K K Wagh College of Pharmacy, Dr Babasaheb Ambedkar Technological University, Raigad, Maharashtra, India

*Address all correspondence to: bedseanjali1980@gmail.com

References

[1] Zeng L, Lin X, Li P, Liu F-Q, Guo H, Li W-H. Recent advances of organogels: From fabrications and functions to applications. Progress in Organic Coatings. 2021;**159**:106417

[2] Rahman M, Hussain A. Lecithin-microemulsion based organogels as topical drug delivery system (TDDS). IJCRR: International Journal of Current Research and Review. 2011;**3**(3):22-33

[3] Sravan B, Kamalakar K, Karuna MSL, Palanisamy A. Studies on organogelation of self assembling bis urea type low molecular weight molecules. Journal of Sol-Gel Science and Technology. 2014;**71**(2):372-379

[4] Cao X, Zhao X, Gao A, Xu R. Organogel formation based on bis-urea derivative. Supramolecular Chemistry. 2014;**26**(10-12):804-808

[5] Behera B, Sagiri SS, Pal K, Srivastava A. Modulating the physical properties of sunflower oil and sorbitan monopalmitate-based organogels. Journal of Applied Polymer Science. 2013;**127**(6):4910-4917

[6] Sagiri SS. Studies on the Synthesis and Characterization of Encapsulated Organogels for Controlled Drug Delivery Applications. Odisha, India: 2014 ethesis published at Department of Biotechnology and Medical Engineering, National Institute of Technology; 2014

[7] Vintiloiu A, Leroux J-C. Organogels and their use in drug delivery – A review. Journal of Controlled Release [Internet].2008;125(3):179-192. Available from: https://www.sciencedirect.com/science/article/pii/S0168365907005391

[8] Jiao T, Wang Y, Zhang Q, Zhou J, Gao F. Regulation of substituent groups on morphologies and self-assembly of organogels based on some azobenzene imide derivatives. Nanoscale Research Letters. 2013;**8**(1):1-8

[9] Sagiri SS, Behera B, Rafanan RR, Bhattacharya C, Pal K, Banerjee I, et al. Organogels as matrices for controlled drug delivery: A review on the current state. Soft Materials. 2014;**12**(1):47-72

[10] Pal A, Dey J. Gelation of organic solvents by N-(n-tetradecylcarbamoyl)-l-amino acids. Supramolecular Chemistry. 2015;**27**(1-2):127-135

[11] Vigato AA, Querobino SM, de Faria NC, de Freitas ACP, Leonardi GR, de Paula E, et al. Synthesis and characterization of nanostructured lipid-poloxamer organogels for enhanced skin local anesthesia. European Journal of Pharmaceutical Sciences. 2019;**128**:270-278

[12] Ibrahim MM, Hafez SA, Mahdy MM. Organogels, hydrogels and bigels as transdermal delivery systems for diltiazem hydrochloride. Asian Journal of Pharmaceutical Sciences. 2013;**8**(1):48-57

[13] Raut S, Bhadoriya SS, Uplanchiwar V, Mishra V, Gahane A, Jain SK. Lecithin organogel: A unique micellar system for the delivery of bioactive agents in the treatment of skin aging. Acta Pharmaceutica Sinica B. 2012;**2**(1):8-15

[14] Jose J, Gopalan K. Organogels: A versatile drug delivery tool in pharmaceuticals. Research Journal of Pharmacy and Technology. 2018;**11**(3):1242-1246

[15] Mujawar NK, Ghatage SL, Yeligar VC. Organogel: Factors and its importance. International Journal

of Biological and Chemical Sciences [Internet]. 2014;4(3):758-773. Available from: https://www.researchgate.net/publication/305359032

[16] Saha S, Shivarajakumar R, Karri VVSR. Pluronic lecithin organogels: An effective topical and transdermal drug delivery system. International Journal of Pharmaceutical Sciences and Research. 2018;**9**(11):4540-4550

[17] Elnaggar YSR, El-Refaie WM, El-Massik MA, Abdallah OY. Lecithin-based nanostructured gels for skin delivery: An update on state of art and recent applications. Journal of Controlled Release. 2014;**180**:10-24

[18] Mehta C, Bhatt G, Kothiyal P. A review on organogel for skin aging. Indian Journal of Pharmaceutical and Biological Research. 2016;**4**(3):28

[19] Sahoo S, Kumar N, Bhattacharya C, Sagiri SS, Jain K, Pal K, et al. Organogels: Properties and applications in drug delivery. Designed Monomers and Polymers. 2011;**14**(2):95-108

[20] Chang C-E, Hsieh C-M, Chen L-C, Su C-Y, Liu D-Z, Jhan H-J, et al. Novel application of pluronic lecithin organogels (PLOs) for local delivery of synergistic combination of docetaxel and cisplatin to improve therapeutic efficacy against ovarian cancer. Drug Delivery. 2018;**25**(1):632-643

[21] Belgamwar VS, Pandey MS, Chauk DS, Surana SJ. Pluronic lecithin organogel. Asian Journal of Pharmaceutics. 2008;**2**(3):134-138

[22] Sharma J, Agrawal D, Sharma AK, Khandelwal M, Aman S. New topical drug delivery system pharmaceutical organogel: A review. Asian Journal of Pharmaceutical Research and Development. 2022;**10**(1):75-78

[23] Charoensumran P, Ajiro H. Controlled release of testosterone by polymer-polymer interaction enriched organogel as a novel transdermal drug delivery system: Effect of limonene/PG and carbon-chain length on drug permeability. Reactive and Functional Polymers. 2020;**148**:104461

[24] Lim PFC, Liu XY, Kang L, Ho PCL, Chan YW, Chan SY. Limonene GP1/PG organogel as a vehicle in transdermal delivery of haloperidol. International Journal of Pharmaceutics. 2006;**311**(1):157-164 Available from: https://www.sciencedirect.com/science/article/pii/S0378517305008690

[25] Scartazzini R, Luisi PL. Organogels from lecithins. The Journal of Physical Chemistry. 1988;**92**(3):829-833

[26] Rees GD, Robinson BH. Microemulsions and organogels: Properties and novel applications. Advanced Materials. 1993;**5**(9):608-619

[27] Jenta TR, Batts G, Rees GD, Robinson BH. Biocatalysis using gelatin microemulsion-based organogels containing immobilized chromobacterium viscosum lipase. Biotechnology and Bioengineering. 1997;**53**(2):121-131

[28] Madamwar D, Thakar A. Entrapment of enzyme in water-restricted microenvironment for enzyme-mediated catalysis under microemulsion-based organogels. Applied Biochemistry and Biotechnology. 2004;**118**(1):361-369

[29] Upadhyay KK, Tiwari C, Khopade AJ, Bohidar HB, Jain SK. Sorbitan ester organogels for transdermal delivery of sumatriptan. Drug Development and Industrial Pharmacy. 2007 Jun;**33**(6):617-625

[30] Murdan S, Gregoriadis G, Florence AT. Novel sorbitan monostearate organogels. Journal of Pharmaceutical Sciences. 1999;**88**(6):608-614

[31] Shah DK, Sagiri SS, Behera B, Pal K, Pramanik K. Development of olive oil based organogels using sorbitan monopalmitate and sorbitan monostearate: A comparative study. Journal of Applied Polymer Science. 2013;**129**(2):793-805

[32] Liao L, Zhong X, Jia X, Liao C, Zhong J, Ding S, et al. Supramolecular organogels fabricated with dicarboxylic acids and primary alkyl amines: Controllable self-assembled structures. RSC Advances. 2020;**10**(49):29129-29138

[33] Couffin-Hoarau A-C, Motulsky A, Delmas P, Leroux J-C. In situ-forming pharmaceutical organogels based on the self-assembly of L-alanine derivatives. Pharmaceutical Research. 2004;**21**(3):454-457

[34] Bonam SP. Preparation and Evaluation of Pluronic Lecithin Organogel Containing Ricinoleic Acid for Transdermal Drug Delivery. Toledo, OH, United States: University of Toledo; 2013

[35] Sreedevi T, Ramya D, Vedha H. An emerging era in topical delivery: Organogels. International Journal of Drug Development and Research. 2012;**4**(2):35-40

[36] Shaikh IM, Jadhav KR, Kadam VJ. Lecithin organogels in enhancing skin delivery of drugs. In: Percutaneous Penetration Enhancers Chemical Methods in Penetration Enhancement. Berlin, Heidelberg: Springer Verlag; 2015. pp. 299-313

[37] Reddy G, Reddy D. Organogels – A Review Introduction. International Journal of Pharmacy & Technology. 2010;**2**(4):584-602

[38] Garg T, Bilandi A, Kapoor B, Kumar S, Joshi R. Organogels: Advanced and novel drug delivery system. International Research Journal of Pharmacy. 2011;**2**(12):15-21

[39] Madathil A, Ramalingam N, Krishna N, Mishahal TM, Ganesan B. Organogel - A Topical Drug Delivery Approach. SSRG International Journal of Pharmacy and Biomedical Engineering. 2021;**8**:1-3

[40] Esposito CL, Kirilov P, Roullin VG. Organogels, promising drug delivery systems: An update of state-of-the-art and recent applications. Journal of Controlled Release. 2018;**271**:1-20

[41] Martinez RM, Rosado C, Velasco MVR, da Lannes SCS, Baby AR. Main features and applications of organogels in cosmetics. International Journal of Cosmetic Science. 2019;**41**(2):109-117

[42] Singh VK, Pramanik K, Ray SS, Pal K. Development and characterization of sorbitan monostearate and sesame oil-based organogels for topical delivery of antimicrobials. AAPS PharmSciTech. 2015;**16**(2):293-305

[43] Kantaria S, Rees GD, Lawrence MJ. Gelatin-stabilised microemulsion-based organogels: Rheology and application in iontophoretic transdermal drug delivery. Journal of Controlled Release. 1999;**60**(2-3):355-365

[44] Murdan S. Organogels in drug delivery. Expert Opinion on Drug Delivery. 2005;**2**(3):489-505

[45] Žinic M, Vögtle F, Fages F. Cholesterol-based gelators. In: Low Molecular Mass Gelator. Vol. 256. Topics in Current Chemistry. 2005. pp. 39-76

[46] Hirst AR, Coates IA, Boucheteau TR, Miravet JF, Escuder B, Castelletto V, et al. Low-molecular-weight gelators:

Elucidating the principles of gelation based on gelator solubility and a cooperative self-assembly model. Journal of the American Chemical Society. 2008;**130**(28):9113-9121

[47] Prathap A, Sureshan KM. Sugar-based organogelators for various applications. Langmuir. 2019;**35**(18):6005-6014

[48] Gioia B, Ghalia N Ben, Kirilov P. "Green" Organogelators: Design and Applications. Research and Reviews: Journal of Pharmacy and Pharmaceutical Sciences. 2018;**7**(1):1-11

[49] Suzuki M, Nigawara T, Yumoto M, Kimura M, Shirai H, Hanabusa K. L-Lysine based gemini organogelators: Their organogelation properties and thermally stable organogels. Organic & Biomolecular Chemistry. 2003;**1**(22):4124-4131

[50] Debnath S, Vanitha G, Bindu HP, Babu NM. Applications of organogels in drug delivery. Indian Journal of Research in Pharmacy and Biotechnology. 2014;**2**(1):976

[51] Wang C, Li Z, Wang X, Wei W, Chen S, Sui Z. Gelation mechanism and microstructure of organogels formed with L-valine dihydrazide derivatives. Colloids and Surfaces A: Physicochemical and Engineering Aspects. 2011;**384**(1-3):490-495

[52] Alsaab H, Bonam SP, Bahl D, Chowdhury P, Alexander K, Boddu SHS. Organogels in drug delivery: A special emphasis on organogels pluronic lecithin. Journal of Pharmacy & Pharmaceutical Sciences. 2016;**19**(2):252-273

[53] Thakur VK, Thakur MK, Voicu SI. Polymer Gels: Perspectives and Applications. Gels Horizons: From Science to Smart Materials. Singapore: Springer; 2018. pp. 419

[54] Gökçe EH, Yurdasiper A, Korkmaz E, Özer Ö. A novel preparation method for organogels: High-speed homogenization and micro-irradiation. AAPS PharmSciTech. 2013;**14**(1):391-397

[55] Pisal S, Shelke V, Mahadik K, Kadam S. Effect of organogel components on in vitro nasal delivery of propranolol hydrochloride. AAPS PharmSciTech. 2004;**5**(4):92-100

[56] Liu H, Wang Y, Han F, Yao H, Li S. Gelatin-stabilised microemulsion-based organogels facilitates percutaneous penetration of Cyclosporin A In Vitro and dermal pharmacokinetics In Vivo. Journal of Pharmaceutical Sciences. 2007;**96**(11):3000-3009

[57] Varshosaz J, Andalib S, Tabbakhian M, Ebrahimzadeh N. Development of lecithin nanoemulsion based organogels for permeation enhancement of metoprolol through rat skin. Journal of Nanomaterials. 2013;**2013**:1-10

[58] Shaikh IM, Jadhav KR, Gide PS, Kadam VJ, Pisal SS. Topical delivery of aceclofenac from lecithin organogels: Preformulation study. Current Drug Delivery. 2006 Oct;**3**(4):417-427

[59] Kumar R, Katare OP. Lecithin organogels as a potential phospholipid-structured system for topical drug delivery: A review. AAPS PharmSciTech. 2005;**6**(2):E298-E310

[60] Goto S, Kawata M, Suzuki T, Kim N-S, Ito C. Preparation and evaluation of Eudragit gels. I: Eudragit organogels containing drugs as rectal sustained-release preparations. Journal of Pharmaceutical Sciences. 1991;**80**(10):958-961

[61] van Esch JH, Feringa BL. New functional materials based on self-assembling organogels: From serendipity

towards design. Angewandte Chemie, International Edition. 2000;**39**(13):2263-2266

[62] Hu B, Yan H, Sun Y, Chen X, Sun Y, Li S, et al. Organogels based on amino acid derivatives and their optimization for drug release using response surface methodology. Artificial Cells, Nanomedicine, and Biotechnology. 2020;**48**(1):266-275

[63] Lim PFC, Liu XY, Kang L, Ho PCL, Chan SY. Physicochemical effects of terpenes on organogel for transdermal drug delivery. International Journal of Pharmaceutics [Internet]. 2008;358(1):102-107. Available from: https://www.sciencedirect.com/science/article/pii/S037851730800149X

[64] Silva PM, Martins AJ, Fasolin LH, Vicente AA. Modulation and characterization of wax-based olive oil organogels in view of their application in the food industry. Gels. 2021;7(1):12

[65] Dave P, Patel D, Raval B. An oral organogel-novel approach for controlled drug delivery system. International Journal of Drug Delivery Technology. 2022;**12**(1):437-445

[66] Motulsky A, Lafleur M, Couffin-Hoarau A-C, Hoarau D, Boury F, Benoit J-P, et al. Characterization and biocompatibility of organogels based on L-alanine for parenteral drug delivery implants. Biomaterials. 2005 Nov;**26**(31):6242-6253

[67] Wang K, Jia Q, Han F, Liu H, Li S. Self-assembled L-alanine derivative organogel as in situ drug delivery implant: Characterization, biodegradability, and biocompatibility. Drug Development and Industrial Pharmacy. 2010;**36**(12):1511-1521

[68] Wang D, Zhao J, Liu X, Sun F, Zhou Y, Teng L, et al. Parenteral thermo-sensitive organogel for schizophrenia therapy, in vitro and in vivo evaluation. European Journal of Pharmaceutical Sciences. 2014;**60**:40-48

[69] El Gendy AM, Jun HW, Kassem AA. In vitro release studies of flurbiprofen from different topical formulations. Drug Development and Industrial Pharmacy. 2002;**28**(7):823-831

[70] Marangoni AG, Garti N. An overview of the past, present, and future of organogels. Edible Oleogels: Structure and Health Implications. Champaign, USA: AOCS Press; 2011. pp. 1-17

[71] Esposito CL, Kirilov P. Preparation, characterization and evaluation of organogel-based lipstick formulations: Application in cosmetics. Gels. 2021;7(3):97

[72] Mosquera Narvaez LE, de MC FLM, Sanches S, Alesa Gyles D, JOC S-J, Ribeiro Costa RM. A review of potential use of amazonian oils in the synthesis of organogels for cosmetic application. Molecules. 2022;**27**(9):2733

Chapter 6

Transdermal Delivery of Drugs for Acute and Chronic Pain

Carlos Miguel López-Mendoza, Ana Jared Tenorio-Salazar and Luz Eugenia Alcántara-Quintana

Abstract

Pain is universal, it contributes substantially to morbidity, mortality, and disability, and is a serious health problem. Acute pain usually lasts less than 7 days, but often lasts up to 30 days, and may recur periodically. Chronic pain, defined as lasting more than 3 months, affects approximately 50 million people and generates costs of $635 billion. The problems related to inadequate pain management are frequent and important, so much so that emphasis has been given to the effective delivery of drugs through the skin. This organ has been studied extensively over the last decade because it is easily accessible and would help to solve the problem. It is evident that there is a need to improve transdermal drug delivery (TDD) as it offers multiple advantages, they are noninvasive, can be self-administered, and provide prolonged release. This chapter recapitulates the history of transdermal drug delivery and focuses on addressing the inadequate management of acute and chronic pain.

Keywords: transdermal drug delivery; chronic pain, acute pain, skin

1. Introduction

The International Association for the Study of Pain (IASP) defines pain as "an unpleasant sensory emotional experience associated with actual or potential tissue damage." It is the most frequent symptom in the medical office, associated with innumerable diseases. Pain negatively affects the patient's quality of life because it is usually poorly tolerated and interferes with daily activities. The presence of pain indicates that something is not working well, the perception is subjective and with a great emotional component. The etiology of pain is not always an easy task and requires an accurate assessment to determine its origin [1, 2]. It is important to recognize that not all pain is the same, so we must distinguish and classify each type of pain. Pain is mainly classified according to its duration as chronic pain, whose commonly accepted definition is "that pain that persists beyond the normal healing time," persists to the original cause, and has more than 3 months of duration. On the other hand, we have acute pain, which is of recent onset and lasts less than 3 months. It is important to distinguish between these two types of pain because their pathophysiology is different, therefore, the treatment is different (**Figure 1**) [1, 3]. Common routes of drug

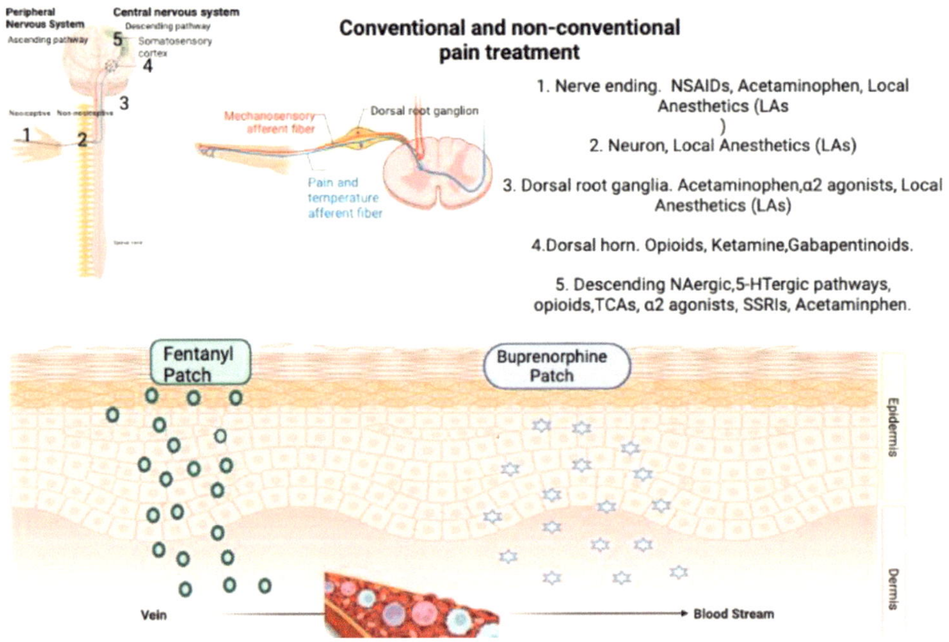

Figure 1.
Conventional and nonconventional pain treatment. The upper part of the figure shows the conventional treatment. The ascending pathway transmits pain and sensory information from the periphery to the brain. Painful stimuli activate primary afferent nociceptors of the mechanosensitive Aδ and C fibers, which send signals to second-order neurons in the spinal cord. This information is transmitted through the spinothalamic tract to tertiary neurons in the thalamus, and pain is perceived in the somatosensory cortex. The descending pathway inhibits pain via noradrenergic/serotonergic neurons and Aβ fibers. Conventional pain treatments and their sites of action (numbers) are shown. The lower part shows the nonconventional treatment, which consists of the application of transdermal patches to control pain. Abbreviation: NSAIDs: Nonsteroidal anti-inflammatory drugs; α2-agonists: α2-adrenergic receptor agonists; TCAs: Tricyclic antidepressants; SSRIs: Selective serotonin reuptake inhibitor.

administration are the oral and parenteral routes. However, their use is limited due to rapid degradation in the stomach. This is just one example as the conventional routes of drug administration could be overcome by using new technologies.

2. History (pain management)

In the 1970s, the first transdermal patches began to be developed, the first one approved being scopolamine, a treatment for motion sickness, which released the drug for 72 hours. Subsequently, nitroglycerin, clonidine, fentanyl, buprenorphine, lidocaine, nicotine, and hormone replacement therapy patches were approved for population management [4, 5].

3. Classification of drugs for acute and chronic pain

Pain is almost universal, and contributes substantially to morbidity, mortality, disability, and health system burden. Acute pain usually lasts less than 7 days, but often lasts up to 30 days, and may recur periodically. Although acute pain usually

Types of pain	Drug administration	Use of a strategy	Use of agents
Mild pain	Administration of paracetamol or NSAIDs	Cognitive-behavioral strategies (relaxation, distraction, etc.)	Physical agents (cold, heat, massage, etc.)
Moderate pain	Administration of low-dose or low-potency Opioids Combinations of paracetamol or NSAIDs with low doses or low-potency opioids	Cognitive-behavioral strategies (relaxation, distraction, etc.)	Physical agents (cold, heat, massage, etc.)
Severe pain	Strong opioid analgesics (intermittent or all day) Continuous infusions of opioid analgesics (e.g., PCA) Neural block (intermittent or continuous) Spinal anesthesia (e.g., epidural anesthesia, intermittent, or continued)	Combined strategies	Not applicable

Table 1.
Pain control options.

resolves quickly, in some cases it may persist until it becomes chronic. Chronic pain, defined as pain lasting more than 3 months, is a serious public health problem in the United States, affecting approximately 50 million people and generating costs of $635 billion. Chronic pain substantially affects physical and mental functioning, reducing productivity and quality of life [6–10].

The American Geriatrics Society Panel on Chronic Pain identified four basic pathophysiologic pain mechanisms that have important implications for choosing pain management strategies [11]. In choosing pain management strategies, it is necessary to adhere to various scales and in this regard, there are several pain measurement scales that help to classify and quantify the magnitude of pain complaints. The results of these scales are also useful for documenting and communicating pain experiences. And in correlation to these scales, the classification of drugs used to treat pain has been made (**Table 1**).

4. Limitations and adverse effects of conventional treatments

The problems related to inadequate pain management are frequent and important. Uncontrolled severe pain can have serious adverse effects on the physical, psychological, emotional, social, and spiritual condition of patients, which has repercussions on daily life activities and leads to economic, labor, and social losses that affect a significant proportion of the population. The functional disability caused by pain is a cause of suffering in patients, their families, and other people close to them. Currently, there are four general categories of analgesic agents frequently used for the most common types of pain: paracetamol, nonsteroidal anti-inflammatory drugs (NSAIDs), and opioids. And one more category such as gamma-aminobutyric acid analogs, gabapentin analogs, and anticonvulsants. However, all of them have adverse effects, Paracetamol has been shown to cause liver damage [10, 11]. NSAIDs are associated with varying degrees of gastrointestinal (GI), cardiovascular, and renal adverse effects. Opioids can cause respiratory depression and cognitive and motor impairment; they can also cause dependence and addiction [12, 13].

5. Transdermal drug delivery systems

The effective delivery of drugs through the skin has been studied during the last decade since the skin is easily accessible. Most compounds are administered with a hypodermic needle, the main limitation of this is pain, needle phobia, and transmission of infectious diseases, so alternatives that circumvent these aspects are sought [14]. However, needles are required to penetrate the skin barrier. The main barrier to delivering a therapeutic agent is the outermost layer of the skin, the stratum corneum (SC). Because of the above, skin permeabilization methods have been developed that offer great advantages over other drug delivery systems [14]. It is evident that there is a need to improve transdermal drug delivery (TDD) as it offers multiple advantages since they are noninvasive and can be self-administered; in addition, it provides prolonged release, i.e., for long periods, and is generally inexpensive when it becomes commercially available. TDD is a painless systemic delivery method, drugs are administered through healthy and intact skin, the drug initially penetrates through the stratum corneum, then passes through the deeper epidermis and dermis without accumulation in the dermal area. When the drug reaches the dermal layer, it becomes available for systemic absorption through dermal microcirculation [14, 15].

First-generation transdermal delivery systems have continued to evolve to reach the clinical setting. They are used in the administration of small, lipophilic, and low-dose drugs. Second-generation delivery systems where we see a different design using chemical enhancers, non-cavitational ultrasound and iontophoresis have also resulted in clinical products. Third-generation delivery systems target the stratum corneum using tools such as microneedles, thermal ablation, microdermabrasion, electroporation, and cavitational ultrasound. Currently, TDDS with microneedle and thermal ablation technology has been developed and is progressing through clinical trials for the delivery of macromolecules, such as insulin and parathyroid hormone [16, 17].

6. Formulation

The basic components of a TDDS include polymer matrix, membrane, drug, penetration enhancers, pressure-sensitive adhesives (PSA), backing laminates, and release coating, the characteristics and examples are enounced in **Table 2**. In **Figure 2** we can observe the composition of each layer that compose different types of TDDS.

7. When to use them or not to use them?

7.1 Transdermal patches are used when

- The patient has intolerant side effects and is unable to take oral medication (dysphagia) and is requesting an alternative method of drug delivery.

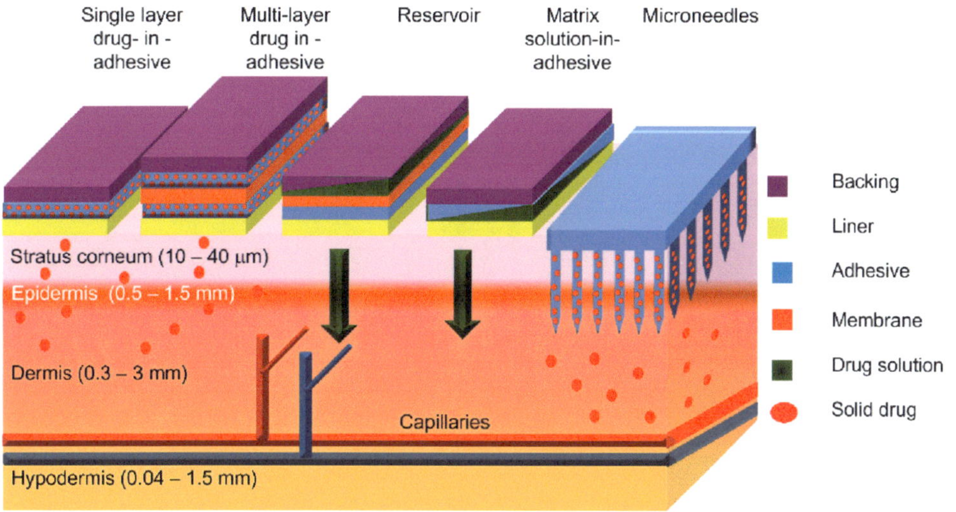

Figure 2.
Types of TDDS. This figure describes the different types of TDDS. Starting from left to right we have single-layer drug-in-adhesive and multi-layer drug-in-adhesive, which are similar in that they contain the drug in the adhesive layer and a solid-state, except for the multilayer, which has a membrane. Finally, we have the microneedle patches, which have penetration to the dermis, with biodegradable needles, from which the solid drug will be released. All these TDDS are intended for the active ingredient to travel to the capillaries between the dermis and the hypodermis.

- Where the confidence of administration may improve pain control. This may be useful in patients with cognitive failure or those who cannot self-medicate for analgesia.

- It can be used in combination with another potentiating strategy that produces a synergistic effect.

7.2 Transdermal patches are not used when

- Cure for acute pain is required.

- When a quick dose is needed.

- When the required dose is equal to 30 mg/24 h or less [23].

8. Advantages, disadvantages, and limitations

In **Table 3** we can observe the advantages and disadvantages of being treated with TDDS.

9. Permeation mechanisms

9.1 Passive (patches)

Patches belong to the first generation of transdermal delivery systems. Significant advances in patch technology have led to their everyday commercial use. Patches are

Component	Description	Desirable characteristics	Examples
Polymer matrix/drug reservoir/membrane	The function of the polymer is to control the release of the active agent. The choice of polymer will depend on the type of drug and the purpose of the device, they must be biocompatible and provide uniform and effective delivery of a drug over the intended lifetime of the product.	Not chemically reactive with the drug. The polymer should not decompose during its shelf life. Molecular weight and physicochemical properties should allow diffusion of the drug at the desired rate. The polymer and its decomposition products must be nontoxic. It must be biocompatible with the skin. The polymer must be easy to make and fabricate into the desired product. It must allow the incorporation of large quantities of the active agent.	PVA PE CE HPMCE ECE PMA PVP PEG
Drug	The physicochemical properties of the drugs must be taken into account since due to skin permeation, it is not possible to use all types of drugs.	Dosage less than 20 mg/day. Half-life in h of 10 or less. Molecular weight less than 400 Log P (octane - water) partition coefficient between 1 and 4. Skin permeability coefficient greater than 0.5 x 10^{-3} cm/h. Not irritating or sensitizing.	Captopril Metoprolol tartrate. Clonidine indapamide Propranolol hydrochloride Carvedilol Verapamil hydrochloride Nifedipine Buprenorphine Fentanyl
Permeation enhancers	Modify the biological barrier of the skin by interacting with the lipids of the stratum corneum to increase permeability to achieve higher concentrations.	They must not be toxic, irritating, or cause allergies. The duration of the effect should be predictable and reproducible. They must not have pharmacological activity with the body. Inert with the drug. They must work in a unidirectional way. Upon removal of the patch, the barrier properties should be reestablished. They must be cosmetically acceptable with an appropriate skin feel.	Terpenes Alcohols Glycols Pyrrolidones Sodium lauryl sulfate Vitamin C Oleic acid Penetratin

Pressure-sensitive adhesives	They are the component that adheres to the skin, through the application of a light force. They form interatomic and intermolecular forces of attraction at the interface, the material should be able to deform under slight pressure and when removed should not leave residues.	High biocompatibility. Good adhesion to oily, moist, wrinkled, and hairy skin. Good environmental resistance (water and humidity) Easy to remove from the skin. High moisture permeability to avoid excessive occlusion and for the drug itself. Not to be reactive with the drug.	Silicone-type adhesive. Polyisobutylene adhesive. Polyacrylate-based adhesive.
Backing laminates	Its purpose is to bind the entire system together and at the same time protect the drug reservoir from exposure to the atmosphere.	Pleasant appearance. Flexibility and need for occlusion. Chemical resistance. Biocompatible. Impermeable to drug and permeation enhancers.	Polyester. Siliconized and aluminized polyethylene terephthalate. Metalized polyester aluminum laminated with polyethylene.
Release liner	The strip prevents loss of the drug that has migrated into the adhesive layer during storage and protects the completed device against contamination.	Chemically inert. Resistant to deformation. Resistant to the environment during shelf life.	Nonocclusive base layer: Paper cloth Occlusive base layer: Polyethylene Polyvinyl chloride Nonstick: Silicone

Table 2.
Characteristics of the TDDS components [18–22].

Advantages	Disadvantages	Limitations
Painless. Noninvasive. They are not bulky and easy to handle and dispose of. Little or no gastrointestinal side effects. It avoids first-pass metabolism. Prevents the degradation of drugs by stomach pH. Self-administration. Increases bioavailability. Reduction of dosing frequency. Alternative for patients with impairment of common routes of administration (oral, IV). Therapy can be terminated when the device is removed.	Contact dermatitis (discontinuation of administration). High cost compared to tablets. You cannot use all drugs. It May cause allergic reactions. A water-lipid solubility between 1 and 3 (log P octanol/water) is necessary for permeation. Only potent drugs are useful candidates for this type of delivery.	They cannot deliver ionic drugs. Cannot have high blood/ plasma drug levels. They cannot be developed for drugs of large molecular size. They cannot be developed if the drug or formulation causes skin irritation. Variation in absorption efficiency at sites other than the skin.

Table 3.
Advantages, disadvantages, and limitations of the TDDS [24–27].

passive permeation systems; drugs diffuse through a membrane from a region of high concentration to areas of low concentration. The rate of diffusion is proportional to the gradient but also depends on the properties of the administered molecule such as solubility, size, degree of ionization, and the adsorption surface. The drug is stored in the polymer and has contact on one side with the impermeable backing and on the other with the adhesive. Some designs employ the drug dissolved in a liquid or gel reservoir, which can simplify formulations [14, 17].

9.2 Active (microneedles)

A simple way to selectively permeabilize the stratum corneum is to pierce it with very short needles. Micro-needle (MN) matrices are minimally invasive drug delivery systems that have the advantage of avoiding the use of hypodermic needles, thus improving patient compliance combines bine the ease of use of a transdermal patch with the effectiveness of hypodermic needle and syringe administration [27, 28].

MN are multiple microscopic projections assembled on a support base or patch; the support must be flexible with characteristics dictated by the properties of the material from which they will be made. Generally ranging from 25 to 2000 μm in height, 50 to 250 μm in width and base, and 1 to 25 μm in tip diameter [27]. The needles must be of adequate length, width, and shape to avoid contact with nerves when inserted into the skin layers. MNs are made of a polymeric matrix, which eventually degrades, thus releasing the therapeutic molecules into the dermis layer in the skin, to reach the blood vessels.

MNs are designed to create transient aqueous conduits through the skin, thus improving the flow of molecules such as low molecular weight heparins, insulin, and vaccines, all without pain [29]. The advantages offered by MN technology are the fact that they do not cause bleeding, eliminate the variability of transdermal dosing of small molecules, minimal risk of introduction of pathogens through MN-induced holes, can be self-administered, and the ease of disposal of MN waste [27, 30].

10. Types of TDDS

See **Figure 2**.

10.1 Single-layer (Unilayer)

It is fabricated with three layers, a temporary liner in the lower, an adhesive in the middle, and a backing on the top, and Is called a Single Layer because the adhesive layer accomplishes two functions: the adhesion in the skin and a container for the active molecule.

10.2 Multilayer

It is like the single layer in that the adhesive layer is the same as the one containing the drug but differs in that it adds another layer of drug-adhesive, usually separated by a membrane. It also has a temporary liner and a permanent backing.

10.3 Reservoir

Unlike the unilayer and multilayer, this system has a separate drug layer. This layer is a liquid compartment containing the drug in solution or suspension separated by an adhesive layer. This patch also has a backing and a temporary liner. Its release kinetics is of zero order.

10.4 Matrix

This system has a drug layer of a semisolid matrix containing a drug solution or suspension. The adhesive layer surrounds the drug layer partially enveloping it.

10.5 Vapor

The adhesive layer of the patch contains oils or another vaporized solution for its release. They release essential oils for more than 6 h to be used in cases of decongestion, other patches improve the quality of sleep and reduce the number of cigarettes in a month [31, 32].

11. Properties affecting delivery

11.1 Physicochemical properties of penetrating molecules

11.1.1 Partition coefficient

A lipid/water partition coefficient, if 1 or greater is required for optimal transdermal permeability.

11.1.2 pH conditions

At moderate pH, the flux of ionizable drugs can be affected by changes in pH that alter the ratio of charged to uncharged species and their transdermal permeability.

11.1.3 Penetrating concentration

At a concentration higher than the solubility, the excess solid drug acts as a reservoir and helps to maintain a constant drug constitution for prolonged periods of time [33, 34].

11.2 Physicochemical properties of the delivery system

11.2.1 Release characteristics

The release mechanisms depend on whether the drug molecules are dissolved or suspended in the systems. Also on the partition coefficient of the drug from the delivery system to the skin and the pH of the vehicle.

11.2.2 Composition of drug systems

The composition of the system (bonded layers, thickness, polymers, and vehicles) not only affects the drug release rate but also the permeability of the stratum corneum due to hydration, making skin lipids or other effects that promote absorption [34].

12. Processing methods

12.1 Patches

Patch manufacturing methods vary according to the type and purpose of the drug to be administered. Transdermal patches are complex pharmaceutical forms, consisting first of an impermeable outer coating layer—whose function is to protect the formulation—a reservoir with the active ingredient and permeation potentiators, an adhesive film that allows its fixation to the skin, and on top of it a removable protective layer that must be removed before application [17, 35].

12.2 Microneedle arrays

The original MN fabrication methods involved clean-room sculpting of silicon-based structures, these have moved to low-cost fabrication methods [36] to make microneedles from metals, silicones, and polymers commonly found in FDA-approved devices. Microneedles offer a high range of possibilities in terms of delivery substances; in several studies, they have been dip-coated with a variety of compounds, including small molecules, proteins, DNA, and virus particles [28, 30, 37].

The shape and geometry of MN are very relevant during design and manufacturing. The needles should be able to be inserted into the skin without damage or breakage and should have the ideal length, width, and shape to avoid contact with nerves [38].

In general, four TDD strategies using MNs. These are solid, coated, soluble, and hollow MNs. Solid MNs are usually fabricated from sheets of solid materials either stainless steel or biocompatible materials, then electropolished. MNs used in antigen delivery studies are prepared as single rows of 5 needles. The needle should have the geometry of a pointed tip on a long elongated shaft, 50 mm thick and 200 mm wide at the base [11].

A recent method in MN fabrication is the use of biocompatible polymers on flexible backings that can be water-soluble. The patches dissolve completely in the skin; because the backing is water-soluble, there is no need to remove the device, ensuring total dissolution and reducing biohazard waste. In addition, due to the flexible backing, the patch can adapt to the skin and localize the insertion forces, this increases the ability of each MN to perforate the SC [18].

High-precision three-dimensional (3D) printing is a novel method of constructing solid micromodels. However, this method is still in its early stages both in the research field and in the pharmaceutical industry [39]. Another recent fabrication method for dissolving needles is the droplet air blowing method. Stamped droplets of polymer can be stretched between two plates. By blowing air between the two plates. The advantages of this method are the mild temperature and pressure requirements and the short fabrication time [40, 41].

13. Application according to the duration of pain

13.1 Acute

The treatment of acute pain should act on the cause, although pain is only a symptom, the sensation of pain should be treated as part of the treatment. In mild pain, the first option is paracetamol. When the pain is moderate, NSAIDs alone or associated with opioids are the best option, and if they are to be avoided, the association of paracetamol with minor opioids is an acceptable alternative. Analgesic escalation prolongs the patient's suffering. Therefore, according to the assessment of pain intensity, prompt action should be taken [42].

For the treatment of acute pain, there are several options available on the market patches, whose active components are ketoprofen, diclofenac, and capsaicin (mild pain); buprenorphine and fentanyl are normally used in cases of chronic pain, in people who are expected to need analgesics 24 hours a day for a long time and who cannot be treated with other drugs.

These options in patch presentation offer advantages such as the patient can apply the patch himself without the need of a professional, the dosage is sustained, does not cause pain, avoids the hepatic metabolism step, is comfortable to wear, and can continue with daily activities.

13.2 Chronic

Chronic pain is associated with malignant (cancer) or nonmalignant conditions. TDDS are effective for the treatment of this type of pain, as the amount of intravenous and oral treatments can become harmful in a short period of time, causing mostly gastrointestinal tract problems. As we have seen throughout this chapter, the advantages of TDDS are also applied to treatment over long periods, although it implies a risk-benefit because these transdermal treatments can also give rise to adverse effects, although of lesser impact.

The approved TDDS for clinical use are composed of opioids, such as buprenorphine (BuTRANS, Transtec) and fentanyl (Duragesic). In addition, these systems can be directed to the elderly patient (> 65 years), we must remember that in these patients the metabolism decreases and the ratio in the body of fat/muscle is altered, consequently the doses of drugs should be decreased, in contrast to those of a young adult, because in the treatment of chronic pain they may suffer from respiratory depression when opioids and non-opioids are delivered by other routes, being an advantage a TDDS of prolonged release. TDDS for chronic pain are contraindicated in the management of acute and postoperative pain [43].

13.2.1 TDDS buprenorphine

Buprenorphine is a semisynthetic opioid, lipophilic in nature, which is intended to provide analgesia. The effect of this drug is of long duration (6–8 h), due to the dissociation of buprenorphine from the mu receptor. On the other hand, the buprenorphine transdermal patch has a slow onset (12–24 h) and a long duration (3 days) [44].

Clinical trials revealed that in patients with moderate to severe chronic pain it is possible to make a treatment switch from weak opioids to transdermal buprenorphine without problems. For patients who respond favorably to this form of release, an example of this is by reporting uninterrupted sleep for more than 6 h compared to a placebo group (without the active ingredient). The mean duration of treatment has been up to 7.5 months of analgesia in 90% of patients. In addition, it has been observed that it can work for neuropathic and nociceptive pain. The safety profile (renal), analgesia over long periods, and is a noninvasive treatment make it an attractive choice for the treatment of chronic pain in elderly patients [44].

Long-term treatment of chronic pain with transdermal buprenorphine has been evaluated for its efficacy and tolerability in cancer and non-cancer patients with moderate to severe pain. Buprenorphine 35 µg/h patches and buprenorphine sublingual tablets (0.2 mg) were used as rescue medication. The duration of maximum participation in cancer patients was 3.4 years and in non-cancer patients 5.7 years. Treatment adherence was 78.7%, with most patients (65.9%) managing their pain with only the patch or taking no more than 1 sublingual tablet daily as adjuvant. Ninety percent of patients reported pain relief and the patch was well tolerated [45].

However, these treatments are not free of adverse effects, since the typical conditions of opioid use have been reported, such as nausea, dizziness, vomiting, constipation, and tiredness, in addition to local effects such as erythema, pruritus and exanthema [44, 45].

13.2.2 TDDS fentanyl

In 1990, the FDA approved the first formulation of an opioid pain medication in a fentanyl-containing patch with a 72 h duration. Fentanyl TDDS is effective and tolerated, forming a depot in the most superficial layers of the skin before entering the microcirculation. Therapeutic concentrations are obtained 12–16 h after patch application and decrease slowly, with a half-life of 16–22 h after patch removal. However, transdermal fentanyl should be used prior to patient sensitization with oral or parenteral opioids to avoid exacerbation of pain or opioid-related adverse effects, which is a disadvantage compared to transdermal buprenorphine [46].

Fentanyl patches were studied in patients with moderate to severe nom-cancer related chronic pain. With starting doses of 12.5 μg/h to be later increased by 12.5 μg/h or 25 μg/h if the average pain score was equal or more than 4 in the first 72 h, the patients' pain relief was notorious, from a scale of 7 out of 10 of pain assessment it was reduced to 2 out of 10, after 12 weeks. In the treatment of soft tissue cancer chronic pain, the relief of pain comes with a 25 μg/h dose patch, within the first 72 h and the severity of pain after treatment decreased significantly [47].

We must remember that these TDDS have their benefit, but also their risk, since the use of this TDDS has reported adverse effects in up to 72% of cases, such as nausea, vomiting and drowsiness. In addition, another effect related to opioids and the transdermal form of the drug is hypoventilation, so its use should be considered in patients with preexisting conditions of lung damage, such as emphysema. Other serious effects of TDDS include cognitive and physical impairments such as confusion or abnormal coordination [48].

14. Conclusions and perspectives

There are several patch options available on the market for the treatment of acute and chronic pain, TDDS are an attractive option because of its advantages over other systems (pills, tablets) and it promotes pharmaceutical adhesion because it is a noninvasive method of dosage and the self-administration. However, considerations must be made in diminishing the secondary and adverse effects of the current ones or to combine new nanosystems for the drug encapsulation for better control of the release. In future outlooks, new smart transdermal delivery systems are being developed that include external stimuli for the release of the drug.

Acknowledgements

We would like to thank CIACYT for their support.

Conflict of interest

The authors declare no conflict of interest.

Notes/thanks/other declaration

We have no further statement to make.

Nomenclature

PVA	Poly (ethylenvinylacetate)
PE	Polyethylene
CE	Cellulose
PMMA	Polymethyl methacrylate
PVP	Polyvinylpyrrolidone
PEG	Polyethylene glycol
HPMCE	Hydroxypropyl methylcellulose
ECE	Ethylcellulose

Author details

Carlos Miguel López-Mendoza, Ana Jared Tenorio-Salazar
and Luz Eugenia Alcántara-Quintana*
Cellular and Molecular Diagnostics Innovation Unit, Coordination
for the Innovation and Application of Science and Technology,
Lomas Segunda Sección, San Luis Potosí, SLP, Mexico

*Address all correspondence to: lealcantara@conacyt.mx

References

[1] Raffaeli W, Arnaudo E. Pain as a disease: An overview. Journal of Pain Research. 2017;**10**:2003. DOI: 10.2147/JPR.S138864

[2] Jackson TP, Stabile VS, McQueen KAK. The Global Burden of Chronic Pain. ASA Newsletter. 2014;**78**:24-27. Available form: https://pubs.asahq.org/monitor/article-abstract/78/6/24/3059/The-Global-Burden-Of-Chronic-Pain?redirectedFrom=fulltext [Accessed: June 11, 2022]

[3] Chen J, Kandle P, Murray I, Fitzgerald L, Sehdev J. Physiology, Pain. 2022 [Internet]. Available from: https://www.ncbi.nlm.nih.gov/books/NBK539789/

[4] Sabatowski R, Schafer D, Kasper M, Radbruch L. Pain Treatmen: A historical overview. Current Pharmaceutical Design. 2004;**10**:1-17. DOI: 10.2174/1381612043452974

[5] Patel D, Chaudhary S, Pamar B, Bhura N. Transdermal drug delivery system: A review. The Pharma Innovation. 2012;**1**:1-10

[6] Institute of Medicine. Relieving Pain in America: A Blueprint for Transforming Prevention, Care, Education, and Research. Washington, DC: The National Academies Press; 2011

[7] Treede RD, Rief W, Barke A, et al. Chronic pain as a symptom or a disease: The IASP classification of chronic pain for the international classification of diseases (ICD-11). Pain. 2019;**160**(1):19-27. DOI: 10.1097/j.pain.0000000000001384

[8] Gaskin DJ, Richard P. The economic costs of pain in the United States. The Journal of Pain. 2012;**13**(8):715-724. DOI: 10.1016/j.jpain.2012.03.009

[9] Dahlhamer J, Lucas J, Zelaya C, Nahin R, Mackey S, DeBar L, et al. Prevalence of Chronic Pain and High-Impact Chronic Pain among Adults. Morbidity and Mortality Weekly Report (MMWR). United States; 2016;**67**(36):1001-1006. DOI: 10.15585/mmwr.mm6736a2

[10] Ferrell BA. Pain management. Clinics in geriatric medicine. 2000;**16**(4):853-874. DOI: 10.1016/s0749-0690(05)70048-3

[11] Blondell RD, Azadfard M, Wisniewski AM. Pharmacologic therapy for acute pain. American Family Physician. 2013;**87**(11):766-772

[12] Bower WA, Johns M, Margolis HS, Williams IT, Bell BP. Population-based surveillance for acute liver failure. The American Journal of Gastroenterology. 2007;**102**(11):2459-2463

[13] National Comprehensive Cancer Network. NCCN Clinical Practice Guidelines in Oncology: Adult Cancer Pain, Version.2.2013. NCCN website. http://www.nccn.org/professionals/physician.gls/f_guidelines_nojava.asp [Accessed: September 12, 2013]

[14] Jeong WY, Kwon M, Choi HE, Kim KS. Recent advances in transdermal drug delivery systems: A review. Biomaterials Research. 2021;**25**(1):1-15. DOI: 10.1186/s40824-021-00226-6

[15] Vargason AM, Anselmo AC, Mitragotri S. The evolution of commercial drug delivery technologies. Nature Biomedical Engineering.

2021;**5**(9):951-967. DOI: 10.1038/s41551-021-00698-w

[16] Rastogi V, Yadav P. Transdermal drug delivery system: An overview. Asian Journal of Pharmaceutics (AJP). 2012;**6**(3):1-10. DOI: 10.1038/s41551-021-00698-w

[17] Prausnitz MR, Langer R. Transdermal drug delivery. Nature Biotechnology. 2008;**26**(11):1261-1268. DOI: 10.1038/nbt.1504

[18] Goswami T, Audett J. Chemistry, manufacturing and controls in passive transdermal drug delivery systems. Therapeutic Delivery. 2015;**6**(9): 1071-1079. DOI: 10.4155/tde.15.57

[19] Yewale C, Tandel H, Patel A, Mista A. Polymers in transdermal drug delivery. In: Mista A, Shahiwala A, editors. Applications of Polymers in Drug Delivery. 2nd ed. United Kingdom: Elsevier; 2021. p. 131-158. DOI: 10.1016/B978-0-12-819659-5.00005-7. Ch 5

[20] Kashmira K, Harsha K. Film forming Systems for Topical and Transdermal Drug Delivery. Asian Journal of Pharmaceutical Sciences. 2017;**12**(6):487-497. DOI: 10.1016/j.ajps.2017.07.004

[21] Lobo S, Sachdeva S, Goswami T. Role of pressure-sensitive adhesives in transdermal drug delivery systems. Therapeutic Delivery. 2016;7(1):33-48. DOI: 10.4155/tde.15.87

[22] Ramadon D, McCrudden M, Courtenay A, et al. Enhancement strategies for transdermal drug delivery systems: Current trends and applications. Drug Delivery and Translations Research. 2022;**12**:758-791. DOI: 10.1007/s13346-021-00909-6

[23] Sudam K, Suresh B. A comprehensive review on: Transdermal drug delivery systems. International Journal of Biomedical and Advance Research. 2016;**7**:147-159. DOI: 10.7439/ijbar

[24] Wang F, Chen Y, Huang Y, Cheng M. Transdermal drug delivery systems for fighting common viral infectious diseases. Drug delivery and translational research. 2021;**11**(4):1498-1508. DOI: 10.1007/s13346-021-01004-6

[25] Shingade G et al. Review on: Recent trend on transdermal drug delivery system. Journal of Drug Delivery and Therapeutics. 2012;**2**(1):1-10. DOI: 10.22270/jddt.v2i1.74

[26] Escobar J et al. Nanocarriers for transdermal drug delivery. Research and Reports in Transdermal Drug Delivery. 2012;**1**(3):1-15. DOI: 10.2147/RRTD.S32621

[27] Dinesh M, Vikas P, Rahul M, Piyush G, Rakesh KT. Cutaneous and transdermal drug delivery: Techniques and delivery. In: Rakesh T, editor. Advances in Pharmaceutical Product Development and Research. 1st ed. United Kingdom: Elsevier; 2019. p. 595-650. DOI: 10.1016/B978-0-12-817909-3.00015-7. Ch 15

[28] Kim Y-C, Park J-H, Prausnitz MR. Microneedles for drug and vaccine delivery. Advanced Drug Delivery Reviews. 2012;**64**(14):1547-1568. DOI: 10.1016/j.addr.2012.04.005

[29] Gupta J, Felner EI, Prausnitz MR. Minimally invasive insulin delivery in subjects with type 1 diabetes using hollow microneedles. Diabetes Technology & Therapeutics. 2009;**11**(6):329-337. DOI: 10.1089/dia.2008.0103

[30] Damiri F, Kommineni N, Ebhodaghe SO, Bulusu R, Jyothi VGSS, Sayed AA, et al. Microneedle-based

natural polysaccharide for drug delivery systems (DDS): Progress and challenges. Pharmaceuticals. 2022;**15**(2):190. DOI: 10.3390/ph15020190

[31] Al H, Khan H, Sarfraz M, Arafat M, Ijaz S, Hameed A. Transdermal patches: Design and current approaches to painless drug delivery. Acta Pharmaceutica. 2019;**69**(2):197-215. DOI: 10.2478/acph-2019-0016

[32] Ahmed S et al. Current trends in polymer microneedle for transdermal drug delivery. International Journal of Pharmaceutics. 2020;**587**:1-15. DOI: 10.1016/j.ijpharm.2020.119673

[33] Singh I, Morris A. Performance of transdermal therapeutic systems: Effects of biological factors. International journal of Pharmaceutical Investigation. 2011;**1**(1):4-9. DOI: 10.4103/2230-973X.76721

[34] Gorzelanny C, Mess C, Schneider SW, Huck V, Brandner JM. Skin barriers in dermal drug delivery: Which barriers have to Be overcome and how can we measure them? Pharmaceutics. 2020;**12**(7):684. DOI: 10.3390/pharmaceutics12070684

[35] Ma K, Jiang W, Wang Y-X, Wang L, Lv Y, Liu J-F, et al. Expert consensus of the Chinese Association for the Study of pain on pain treatment with the transdermal patch. World Journal of Clinical Cases. 2021;**9**(9):2110. DOI: 10.12998/wjcc.v9.i9.2110

[36] Henschke N, Kamper J, Maher C. The Epidemiology and Economic Consequences of Pain. Mayo Clinic proceedings. 2015;**90**(1):139-147. DOI: 10.1016/j.mayocp.2014.09.010

[37] Gill HS, Prausnitz MR. Coated microneedles for transdermal delivery. Journal of Controlled Release. 2007;**117**(2):227-237. DOI: 10.1016/j.jconrel.2006.10.017

[38] Park J-H, Allen MG, Prausnitz MR. Polymer microneedles for controlled-release drug delivery. Pharmaceutical Research. 2006;**23**(5):1008-1019. DOI: 10.1007/s11095-006-0028-9

[39] Wu M, Xia T, Li Y, Wang T, Yang S, Yu J, et al. Design and fabrication of r-hirudin loaded dissolving microneedle patch for minimally invasive and long-term treatment of thromboembolic disease. Asian Journal of Pharmaceutical Sciences. 2022;**17**(2):284-297. DOI: org/10.1016/j.ajps.2022.02.005

[40] Schoellhammer CM, Blankschtein D, Langer R. Skin permeabilization for transdermal drug delivery: Recent advances and future prospects. Expert Opinion on Drug Delivery. 2014;**11**(3):393-407. DOI: 10.1517/17425247.2014.875528

[41] Kim JD, Kim M, Yang H, Lee K, Jung H. Droplet-born air blowing: Novel dissolving microneedle fabrication. Journal of Controlled Release. 2013;**170**(3):430-436. DOI: 10.1016/j.jconrel.2013.05.026

[42] Blanco-Tarrío E. Acute pain management. Semergen-Family Medicine. 2010;**36**(7):392-398. DOI: 10.1016/j.semerg.2010.05.003

[43] Vadivelu N, Hines RL. Management of chronic pain in the elderly: Focus on transdermal buprenorphine. Clinical Interventions in Aging. 2008;**3**(3): 421-430. DOI: 10.2147/cia.s1880

[44] Sittl R. Transdermal buprenorphine in the treatment of chronic pain. Expert Review of Neurotherapeutics. 2005 May;**5**(3):315-323. DOI: 10.1586/14737175.5.3.315

[45] Rudolf Likar, Hubertus Kayser, Reinhard Sittl. Long-term management of chronic pain with transdermal buprenorphine: A multicenter, open-label, follow-up study in patients from three short-term clinical trials. Clinical Therapeutics. 2006;**28**(6):943-952. ISSN 0149-2918. DOI: 10.1016/j.clinthera.2006.06.012 (https://www.sciencedirect.com/science/article/pii/S0149291806001482)

[46] Kornick CA, Santiago-Palma J, Moryl N, et al. Benefit-risk assessment of transdermal fentanyl for the treatment of chronic pain. Drug-Safety. 2003;**26**: 951-973. DOI: 10.2165/00002018-200326130-00004

[47] Park JH, Kim JH, Yun SC, et al. Evaluation of efficacy and safety of fentanyl transdermal patch (Durogesic®D-TRANS) in chronic pain. Acta Neurochirurgica. 2011;**153**:181-190. DOI: 10.1007/s00701-010-0785-4

[48] Hemati K, Zaman B, Hassani V, Imani F, Dariaie P. Efficacy of fentanyl transdermal patch in the treatment of chronic soft tissue cancer pain. Anesthesiology and Pain Medicine. 2015;**5**(1):e22900. DOI: 10.5812/aapm.22900

Chapter 7

Mesoporous Silica Based Cancer Theranostic: A Modern Approach in Upcoming Medicine

Ajinkya Pote, Vikas Ahirrao and Vishal Pande

Abstract

In case cancers are located deep inside the body and are very tough to diagnose, diagnostic tools like MRI/CT scans can be employed to detect these cancers. The major challenge in such cases is the delivery of MRI active agents or visualizing agents to the target site. In this context we will discuss different mesoporous nanoparticles that can be employed to target the tissue at a specific location, its functionalization to reach the target site (Folic acid), different simple dyes as well as specific dyes which offer theranostic functionality. The nanoparticles like mesoporous silica nanoparticles offer the possibility to load therapeutic and diagnostic agents. Its surface allow multiple functionalization and conjugations which offer target specific delivery of these agents. Moreover we will also overview different modern drug delivery inventions for offering theranostic application.

Keywords: cancer, challenges, diagnosis, mesoporous silica nanoparticle, theranostic application

1. Introduction

Sporadic and wild cell development is profoundly connected with malignant growth. With metastasis and intrusion-related to harmful phenotypic conduct, malignancy forcefully assaults different territories of the human body and is broadly accepted to be one of the most dependable illnesses throughout the world Over the previous decade, the rate and passing rate related to disease have risen pointedly. As indicated by the 2015 World Health Organization figures, malignancy is one of the central reasons for death in industrialized countries. In unindustrialized countries, it is second just to cardiovascular illness as the primary driver of death. It is Expectable that by 2020, the number of progress from a disease will include 13% of the all-out through the world. Current threatening cell treatment models, for example, chemotherapy, medical procedure, photodynamic treatment (PDT), and radiotherapy, are fit for dragging out a patient's life somewhat and helping them to live more. In any case, radiotherapy has hindering impacts, for example, the danger of minor threat at the uncovered zone, and it can venture to such an extreme as to harm live and solid tissues. Chemotherapy is portrayed by the utilization of an assortment of chemotherapeutic specialists to slaughter disease cells and stop its expansion.

IntechOpen

Acute Lymphocytic Leukemia	Basal and Squamous Cell Skin Cancer	Brain and Spinal Cord Tumors in Adults	Gallbladder Cancer	Nasal Cavity and Paranasal Sinuses Cancer	Malignant Mesothelioma
Acute Myeloid Leukemia	Bile Duct Cancer	Brain and Spinal Cord Tumors in Children	Gastrointestinal Neuroendocrine (Carcinoid) Tumors	Nasopharyngeal Cancer	Merkel Cell Skin Cancer
Adrenal Cancer	Bladder Cancer	Breast Cancer	Gastrointestinal Stromal Tumor (GIST)	Neuroblastoma	Multiple Myeloma
Anal Cancer	Bone Cancer	Breast Cancer in Men	Gestational Trophoblastic Disease	Non-Hodgkin Lymphoma	Myelodysplastic Syndromes
Cervical Cancer	Brain and Spinal Cord Tumors in Adults	Endometrial Cancer	Melanoma Skin Cancer	Oral Cavity and Oropharyngeal Cancer	Osteosarcoma
Chronic Lymphocytic Leukemia (CLL)	Brain and Spinal Cord Tumors in Children	Esophagus Cancer	Kaposi Sarcoma	Pituitary Tumors	Pancreatic Cancer
Chronic Myeloid Leukemia (CML)	Hodgkin Lymphoma	Ewing Family of Tumors	Kidney Cancer	Prostate Cancer	Pancreatic Neuroendocrine Tumor (NET)
Salivary Gland Cancer	Skin Cancer	Small Intestine Cancer	Soft Tissue Sarcoma	Stomach Cancer	Testicular Cancer
Chronic Myelomonocytic Leukemia (CMML)	Ovarian Cancer	Eye Cancer (Ocular Melanoma)	Retinoblastoma	Rhabdomyosarcoma	Penile Cancer
Vaginal Cancer	Vulvar Cancer	Waldenstrom Macroglobulinemia	Wilms Tumor	Thyroid Cancer	Uterine Sarcoma

Table 1.
Types of cancers.

Various chemotherapeutic specialists are not cell-explicit and, in this way, are fit for pulverizing ordinary cells and further adding to perpetual fundamental issues. Notwithstanding not being cell-explicit, the aggravation of multidrug obstruction, displayed by most malignant growth cells, acts as a genuine restriction and adds to the low restorative list of chemotherapy. One promising, rising order is nanomedicine, which incorporates nanotechnology and biomedicine [1]. Nanomedicine has incredible potential for growing the therapy of different infirmities, including diabetes, tissue designing, and heart sicknesses, just as extraordinary possible applications in disease theranostics. The fast development of novel nanomaterials has become an extraordinary stage for defeating the unfriendly impacts of chemotherapy, even without the most punctual stage determination of malignancy. In this way, wonderful methodologies have been taken to create nanomaterials for malignancy theranostics. Bio-imaging combined with malignant growth treatment has been shown by Loo et al., who created nanoshells focused on the insusceptible framework to recognize and slaughter bosom disease cells. Different investigations have likewise made monstrous forward leaps. Similarly, mesoporous silica nanomaterials (MSNs) have extraordinary potential as functionalized nanoparticles [2]. An early case of their utility included a cycle in which folic acid (FA) was combined, and changed MSNs were utilized for a focused exchange of the water-safe anticancer prescription camptothecin. In entirety, the examination performed has uncovered that mesoporous silica nanoplexes have significant in vitro and in vivo disease obliteration abilities, and they have applications in imaging and malignant growth treatment at the same time as the investigation into nanomaterials keeps on rising, nanomedicine as a field of study is anticipated to serve a significant part in malignancy analysis and treatment. Silica is one of the pinnacle regular assets accessible on earth and assumes a significant part in medication, primarily regarding human skin and bones, etc. Sorted by the FDA as for the most part perceived as protected generally recognized as safe (GRAS), silicon dioxide is commonly utilized as a food added substance and in the beauty care products and drug businesses. Due to the part of silica in soothing biosafety concerns and the simplicity of the cycles engaged with the manufacture of silica, silica nanomaterials assume an extremely indispensable function in biomedical investigations. In the course of the most recent decade, mesoporous nanomaterials have pulled in developing consideration in the fields of optical imaging, magnetic resonance imaging (MRI), photodynamic treatment, and medication conveyance. MSNs show more wide-running possibilities than other medication conveyance frameworks and offer empowering justification for simultaneous disease determination and treatment, just as medication (**Table 1**) [3, 4].

2. Introduction of cancer including types and treatment available

Body is made up of millions of tiny cells, each of which is a separate living organism. Usually, each cell attaches to the other, including the tissues and organs of your body. One way in which this interaction occurs is seen in the way your cells reproduce. Normal cells in the body grow and divide over time and then stop growing and dividing. Thereafter, they present themselves as needed to replace defective or dying cells. Cancer occurs when the cell production process is out of control. In other words, cancer is a disease characterized by uncontrolled, irregular and irregular cell division. Unlike normal cells, cancer cells continue to grow and divide throughout life, replicating themselves into more dangerous cells [5].

The abnormal growth and differentiation seen in cancer cells is caused by damage to these DNA in cells. There are various ways in which cellular DNA can be altered and gets defective. For example, environmental factors, such as exposure to smoke can trigger a series of events leading to change in normal cellular DNA and that causes cancer. Alternatively, faulty DNA can be inherited from your parents.

As cancer cells divide and multiply, they often form a combination of cancer cells called tumors. Tissues cause many symptoms of cancer by suppressing, crushing, and destroying non-cancerous cells and tissues The currently available treatment for carcinoma is surgery, radiation therapy, chemotherapy, immunotherapy to treat cancer, targeted therapy, Hormone therapy, Stem cell transplant, precision medicine [5].

Surgery: The surgery may be carried out by giving either local anesthesia, regional anesthesia, general anesthesia and physical giving cut and removing the tumor. The other options available are Cryosurgery, Laser, Hyperthermia, Photodynamic Therapy.

Radiation therapy: It is a cancer therapy that involves the use of focused radiation beams to destroy cancer cells and shrink tumors. External beam treatment is the most prevalent method of radiation therapy. A equipment that focuses high-energy radiation beams onto cancer cells is used in this sort of treatment. Radiation may be aimed to precise locations with this device.

Chemotherapy: Chemotherapy causes cell division to be disrupted. The nucleus, located at the centre of each live cell, is the cell's control centre. It is made up of chromosomes, which carry genes. Each time a cell divides into two to generate new cells, these genes must be duplicated exactly. Chemotherapy causes genetic harm in the nucleus of cells. Some medications cause harm to cells when they divide. Some cause harm to cells when they duplicate all of their DNA before splitting. Chemotherapy has a lower risk of harming cells that are dormant, such as most normal cells. Chemotherapy medicines are frequently used in combination. This will include medications that harm cells at various phases of the cell division process.

Immunotherapy: Immunotherapy is a form of cancer treatment which helps combat cancer in your immune system. Your body is supported by the immune system to prevent viruses and other diseases. It is composed of lymph system white blood cells and organs and tissues. Immunotherapy is a biological form of treatment. Biological therapy is a method of medicine used to cure cancer by using medicines created from living organisms.

Targeted Therapy: Targeted therapies are either small-molecule drugs or monoclonal antibodies. The functionalised nanoparticles are able to deliver the molecules to the targeted sites, i.e., API/another chemotherapeutics.

Hormone therapy: it is a form of systemic therapy—a way of administering drugs so they travel throughout the body, rather than being delivered directly to the cancer—that works to add, block or remove hormones from the body to slow or stop the growth of cancer cells.

Stem Cell Transplant: A stem cell transplant (also known as a bone marrow transplant) is a procedure in which defective or cancerous bone marrow is replaced with new, healthy bone marrow cells. A stem cell transplant may be used to treat leukemia and lymphoma, cancers that affect the blood and lymphatic system.

There are two types of stem cell transplantation:

Autologous stem cell transplant:

Healthy cells are isolated from bone marrow of patients. The bone marrow taken from the person initially frozen till it is ready to use. Meanwhile, patient prepare their body for conditioning regimen for transplant. In this process he may receive high dose of multiple therapies and these treatments destroys cancer cells but they also kill bone marrow cells. The patient is injected with their own stored blood stem cells. These cells restore ability to produce blood cells in body.

Allogeneic stem cell transplant:

In this type, the donor stem cells are injected in patient when he has undergone chemotherapy. The allogeneic stem cell transplantation can help fight cancer directly. The cells donated by person they generate new immune response in patient (they find and kill cancer cells) this immune response generated by new cells is better than original immune cells [3].

3. Major challenges in treatment of cancer

Medical services foundation in developing business sectors, nonetheless, has not stayed up with the ascent in non-transferable maladies, particularly malignancy. Verifiable wellbeing needs, for example, adolescence and transferable maladies remain needs, in front of malignancy, ceaseless infections, and different ailments of maturing. Given restricted assets and fixed government medical care financial plans, general wellbeing frameworks face extensive difficulties in conveying convenient finding and therapy to malignancy patients [1].

3.1 Challenges for targeted therapies in cancer treatment

The advancing our comprehension of the sub-atomic pathway that direct cell development, apoptosis, angiogenesis and metastasis, and the correspondence or cross-talk between these transformed pathways and receptors [6].

Several critical steps need to be realized in the application of targeted therapies in malignant growth control:

Developing clinically helpful prognostic markers to distinguish individual requiring treatment.

Developing prescient markers that distinguish and select people who will profit most from these treatments.

Avoiding treatment in those improbable to react or in danger of inadmissible harmfulness.

Combining operators that target distinctive key pathways.

Combining specialists with regular treatments.

Developing techniques to conquer procured obstruction [7].

Clinical preliminaries are fundamental and assume a key function intending to this issue.

The trublesomes of the targeted therapy is that the results are not always as expected. However the assurance of targeted therapy are self-evident, its challenges are not as conspicuous. To accomplish the promises and commensurate the challenges of targeted therapy, one needs to look at the basics of cancer biology. As a initiators, one has to unfold the mystery of driver mutations, intra-tumoural heterogeneity and cancer subtypes.

3.2 Challenges involved in cancer immunotherapy

The approach to cancer immunotherapy involves harnessing the specificity and killing mechanisms of the immune system to target and extirpate malignant cells.

To apply immunotherapies to a larger demography of patients, more conserved indicators expressed on the surface of tumor cells must be found. The purpose of active immunotherapy is to target a particular sequence known as "neoantigens" or tumor-specific antigens that is only expressed on tumor cells (TSA). However, many of the antigens found on tumors are also found on healthy cells, making any therapy including a nontumor specific antigen deadly to healthy cells. Identifying TSA targets for immunotherapy would almost certainly result in improved treatment results with minimum harm to healthy cells. The cancer-testis antigens (CTAs), which are expressed more easily on cancer cells than on healthy ones, are one example of a possible target. Another feature of these antigens is that they generate a strong immunological response. Cancer stem cells, a secretive subgroup of the tumor that contributes to its ability to self-renew continuously even after therapeutic intervention, also express CTAs. Identifying additional markers would therefore assist to overcome the problems given by tumor heterogeneity, since the likelihood of targeting more than one kind of cell would be improved if the host immune cells were "trained" to detect several antigens and launch a vigorous attack on the entire tumor [8].

Due to the development of metabolomics and imaging detection technology, the complex metabolic changes that are involved in the occurrence and development of tumors have become increasingly clear. Metabolic control is a potent weapon that the tumor can employ to break through the growth barrier, as well as a basic activity throughout tumor growth. The tumor's flexible and complex metabolic patterns can promote tumor adaptation to different microenvironments while also contributing to the secretion of inflammatory factors that inhibit immune cell function in the microenvironment and, as a result, interfere with normal metabolism in the body, creating an environment that promotes tumor cell malignancy. Furthermore, tumor cells and normal cells overlap metabolic pathways, making it challenging to intervene in tumor metabolism without impacting normal cells. As a result, there are still several challenges in the targeted therapy of tumor metabolism, as well as numerous concerns in the field of tumor metabolic control. Active peptides typically have 2 to 30 amino acid residues and have beneficial properties such as strong curative effects, reduced side effects, small molecular weights, and easy absorption, which enable them to specifically bind to tumor tissues and interact with tumor growth-related and metastasis-related signal transduction molecules to inhibit tumor growth and metastasis and promote apoptosis in tumor cells. The PI3K/AKT/mTOR, AMPK, STAT3, TRAIL death receptor, and NF-κB signaling pathways are all implicated in tumor metabolism and can be targeted using bioactive peptides. Polypeptide medicines conceived and developed for targeted intervention in signaling pathways are meant to give improved options for treating linked clinical disorders based on this understanding [8].

4. Method for diagnosis of cancer

Malignant growth conclusion includes the different strategies and methods used to recognize or affirm the presence of disease. Finding normally includes an assessment of the patient's history, clinical assessments, survey of research facility test results and radiological information, and minute assessment of tissue tests got by biopsy or fine-needle aspiration. The illness at the beginning phase, when it has a high potential for a fix [9]. Intercessions are accessible which allows the early identification and successful treatment of around 33% of cases.

The early discovery suggests the determination of disease at a beginning phase in its turn of events and is in this way for the most part expected to bring about enhancements intolerant results utilizing traditional treatment procedures. Screening

DOI: http://dx.doi.org/10.5772/intechopen.105447

is a term regularly utilized for approaches that encourage early malignant growth recognition. Screening innovations must be fit for distinguishing little tumors at the beginning phase. Critically, they ought to recognize tumors at a phase when they can be restored by medical procedure alone or when they are more receptive to treatment, subsequently improving patient mortality and bleakness.

Some are the systems which contribute to the analysis of malignant growth

1. Discovery of Novel Molecular Markers for Early Detection

2. Novel Germ-Line Markers of Risk

3. Tissue-Specific Markers of Early Carcinogenesis and carcinogenesis Risk

4. Serum Mark

5. Circulating Tumor and Other Cells

6. Novel Molecular Imaging Approaches

4.1 Molecular (sub-atomic) diagnosis of cancer

Sub-atomic analysis reveals the various changes that happen during the change of an ordinary cell to a tumor cell and catches this data as articulation designs. Mechanically printed microarrays, Real-time PCR, and mi RNAs are generally utilized procedures for estimating this articulation example and help analysts to separate between a typical and a diseased cell. Sub-atomic conclusion through proteomics utilizes surface improved laser desorption/ionization season of flight mass spectrometry and peptide receptors in the planning of protein designs that are associated with harmful development. Nanoscale gadgets quantum spots and carbon nano-cylinders can be promising nano-instruments for compelling estimation of danger. Every one of these methods offers an extraordinary guarantee for altering the finding of disease [10].

4.1.1 Malignant growth diagnosis and nanotechnology

Malignant growth nanotechnology is an interdisciplinary territory of examination which covers a tremendous and various cluster of gadgets like nano-vectors for the focused on the conveyance of anticancer medications and imaging contrast specialists. Nanotechnology is a developing science that can be effectively utilized for malignant growth conclusions in the future. Nanotechnology has developed with wide applications for sub-atomic imaging, sub-atomic determination, and focused on the treatment of malignancy. It assumes a significant function in understanding the objective of identifying changing cell populaces right on time by in vivo imaging or ex vivo investigation. This permits the suitable mix of operators to be picked (in light of exact natural data on the tumor), focusing of these specialists (while keeping away from organic hindrances) to the early disease sores to dispose of or contain them without security impacts on sound tissue, and observing the treatment impact progressively [10].

The essential justification associated with disease nanotechnology is that nanometer-sized particles, for example, semiconductor quantum specks and iron oxide nanocrystals, have optical, attractive, or basic properties that are not accessible from atoms or mass solids. At the point when connected with tumor focusing on ligands, for example, monoclonal antibodies, peptides, or little atoms, these nanoparticles can be utilized to target tumor antigens (biomarkers) just as tumor vasculatures with high fondness and particularity [10]. In the size scope of 5–100 nm breadth, nanoparticles additionally have huge surface regions and utilitarian gatherings for forming to different indicative (e.g., optical, radioisotopic, or attractive) and helpful (e.g., anticancer) specialists. With negligible malignancy cell test readiness, substrate authoritative to even a few antibodies creates a quantifiable change in the gadget's conductivity, prompting a 100-overlap increment in affectability over current indicative methods.

Nanoscale cantilevers, minute, adaptable pillars taking after a column of plunging sheets, are fabricated utilizing semiconductor lithographic strategies. These can be covered with atoms fit for restricting explicit substrates-DNA corresponding to a particular quality grouping, for instance. Such micron-sized gadgets, involving numerous nanometer-sized cantilevers, can recognize single atoms of DNA or protein. Quantum dabs, nanoscale gems of a semiconductor material, for example, cadmium selenide, are another promising nanoscale instrument for research center diagnostics. Nanowires and nano cantilever exhibits are among the main methodologies a work in progress for the early discovery of precancerous and threatening injuries from organic liquids [10, 11].

These improvements raise energizing open doors for customized oncology in which hereditary and protein biomarkers are utilized to analyze and treat malignant growth dependent on the atomic profiles of individual patients [11].

5. Nanoparticle as targeted drug delivery system

Nanotechnology is a quickly extending field, including the advancement of man-made materials in the 5–200 nanometer size range. This measurement tremendously surpasses that of standard natural particles, yet it's lower run moves toward that of numerous proteins and organic macromolecules. In the logical world, the expression "nano" is, nonetheless, to some degree uncertain since it does not assign similar reality for physicists, scientific expert and researcher [12].

Nanorechnology as a rule and nanoparticles specifically have upset the organization of medication. It includes the designing of utilitarian framework at the sub-atomic scale. Such framework are described by remarkable physical, optical and electronic highlights that are appealing for diciplines going from materials science to biomedicine. By ideals of their exceptional physicochemical properties, nanoparticles have indicated guarantee in conveying a scope of particles to wanted destinations in the body. To create more secure and more compelling remedial nanoparticles, analyst have planned novel multifunctional nanoparticle stage for cell/tissue-explicit focusing on, continued or set off medication conveyance, co-conveyance of synergistic medication blend [13].

Nanotechnology is a promising logical way to deal with production, design and manufacture materials, for example, nanoparticles whose size extents between 1 and 1000 nm scale. Their minuscule size, huge surface territory to volume proportion and potential to functionalize their surface give nanoparticles phenomenal physico-concoction properties for their different applications. Nanoparticles have been widely investigated for analytic and remedial applications in clinical and drug industry to fix infections, for example, malignant growth [14].

The essential objectives for examination of nano-bio-innovations in drug conveyance include:

- More specific drug focusing on and conveyance
- Reduction in harmfulness while keeping up restorative impacts
- Greater security and biocompatibility
- Faster improvement of new safe prescriptions

Nanoparticles stacked with the helpful medication can be moved to infection site for focused medication conveyance utilizing following strategies: [15].

1. Active targeting
2. Passive targeting
3. Physical targeting

Active targeting: it includes adjusting the nanoparticle surface by restricting ligands, for example, antibodies and proteins onto the outside of nanoparticle so as to build their take-up by target site. Little size, morphology and electrochemical properties of nanoparticles impact the improved penetration maintenance impact, consequently expanding the capacity of tumor cells to assimilate the nanoparticles contrasted with the ordinary cells. Thus the nanoparticles can be latently focused to the site [15, 16].

Passive targeting: EPR effect became a golden standard in the design of passive tumor-targeted systems. This effect is mostly depends on intrinsic tumor biology and in particular (1) the rate of angiogenesis and lymphangiogenesis, (2) the degree of perivascular tumor growth and the density of the stromal response and, (3) pressure inside the tumor. All the mentioned factors provides a physicochemical characteristic of nanocarriers which will determine its drug delivery efficiency [15, 16].

Physical targeting: Utilizes outside upgrades to direct the nanoparticle to the objective site. The outer boosts additionally control the medication discharge measure. For instance, in the event of photo-thermal treatment light is utilized while in attractive hyperthermia treatment, attractive field is utilized to manage the nanoparticles to the objective site [16].

The drug is either covalently bonded to or physically entrapped in the polymer matrix, depending on the technique of manufacture of polymeric-based drug carriers [17]. The resultant products might be capsules (polymeric nanoparticles or polymer–drug conjugates), polymeric micelles with an amphiphilic core/shell, or hyperbranched macromolecules.

Albumin, chitosan, and heparin are all naturally occurring polymers that have been utilized to carry DNA, oligonucleotides, and proteins, as well as medicines. Recently, serum albumin has been employed as a carrier in the creation of paclitaxel nanoparticles [nanometer-sized albumin-bound paclitaxel, which has been used in the clinic to treat metastatic breast cancer] [18].

Polyamidoamine dendrimer, which was conjugated with cisplatin, is the most extensively employed dendrimer as a scaffold [18]. Dendrimers' highly changeable surface allows them to be conjugated with many molecules at once, such as imaging contrast agents, targeting ligands, or therapeutic medicines, resulting in a dendrimer-based multifunctional drug delivery system [19].

6. Special emphasis on mesoporous silica nanoparticles

Various nanodevices have been accounted like carbon nanotubes, quantum specks, and polymeric micelles, and so on in the field of nanotechnology. In the current situation, mesoporous nanoparticles are developing for their notable medication convey and focusing on purposes. Verifiably, Kresge et al. have portrayed a method for joining sol–gel chemistry with liquid crystal line templating to develop ordered porous molecular sieves characterized by periodic arrangements of uniformly sized mesopores (distance across between 2 nm and 50 nm) consolidated inside an indistinct silica matrix. Mesoporous silica nanoparticles (MSNs) have gotten obvious as a promising and novel medication delivery agent because of their one-of-a-kind mesoporous structure that saving a degree of synthetic solidness, surface usefulness and biocompatibility guarantee the controlled delivery, and target drug delivery of an assortment of API particles [20]. Mesoporous silica materials were found in 1992 by the Mobile Oil Corporation have gotten extensive consideration because of their boss literary properties like, high surface territory, enormous pore volume, tuneable pore diameter, and tuneable pore size distribution. Low toxicity and high loading limit of drug make Mesoporous silica nanoparticles, superior in utilization for controlled and target drug delivery. Essentially, silica is broadly present in nature in contrast with other metal oxides like titanium and iron oxides it has nearly better biocompatibility. The mesoporous type of silica has one-of-a-kind properties, especially in loading of drug, nanoparticles at high amounts, and in the resulting delivery. Because of solid Si-O bond, silica-based mesoporous nanoparticles are steadier to outside reaction, for example, degradation and mechanical stress when contrasted with niosomes, liposomes, and dendrimers which restrain the need of any outer adjustment in the amalgamation of MSNs (**Figures 1** and **2**) (**Table 2**) [25, 26].

6.1 Biocompatibility, biodegradability, toxicity and safety of MSNPs

To be useful for biomedical purposes, any nanomaterial must qualify for regulatory criteria about its biosafety without toxicity. Reasonable evidence on the in vivo toxicity assessment of nanomaterials in animal and human models is needed in this context. Criticality is specifically related to the toxicity and clearance of the MSNs with regard to size, shape, porosity, surface area and charge and chemical functionality. Two scientists, Lin and Haynes, analyzed the impact of various particle sizes of MSNPs varying from 25 to 225 nm by hemolysis testing of red blood cells (RBCs), which revealed a higher percentage of haemolysis found in smaller particle sizes of MSNPs in comparison to larger particles presumably due to the higher surface area [4, 27]. It has been stated in the literature that MSU-2 and MCM-41 are biocompatible when tested against non-cancer CHO cell line model [28]. The toxicological profiles of bare/native MSNPs on animal models were also tested by some investigators and high susceptibility was observed on reticuloendothelial systems, rendering them undesirable for

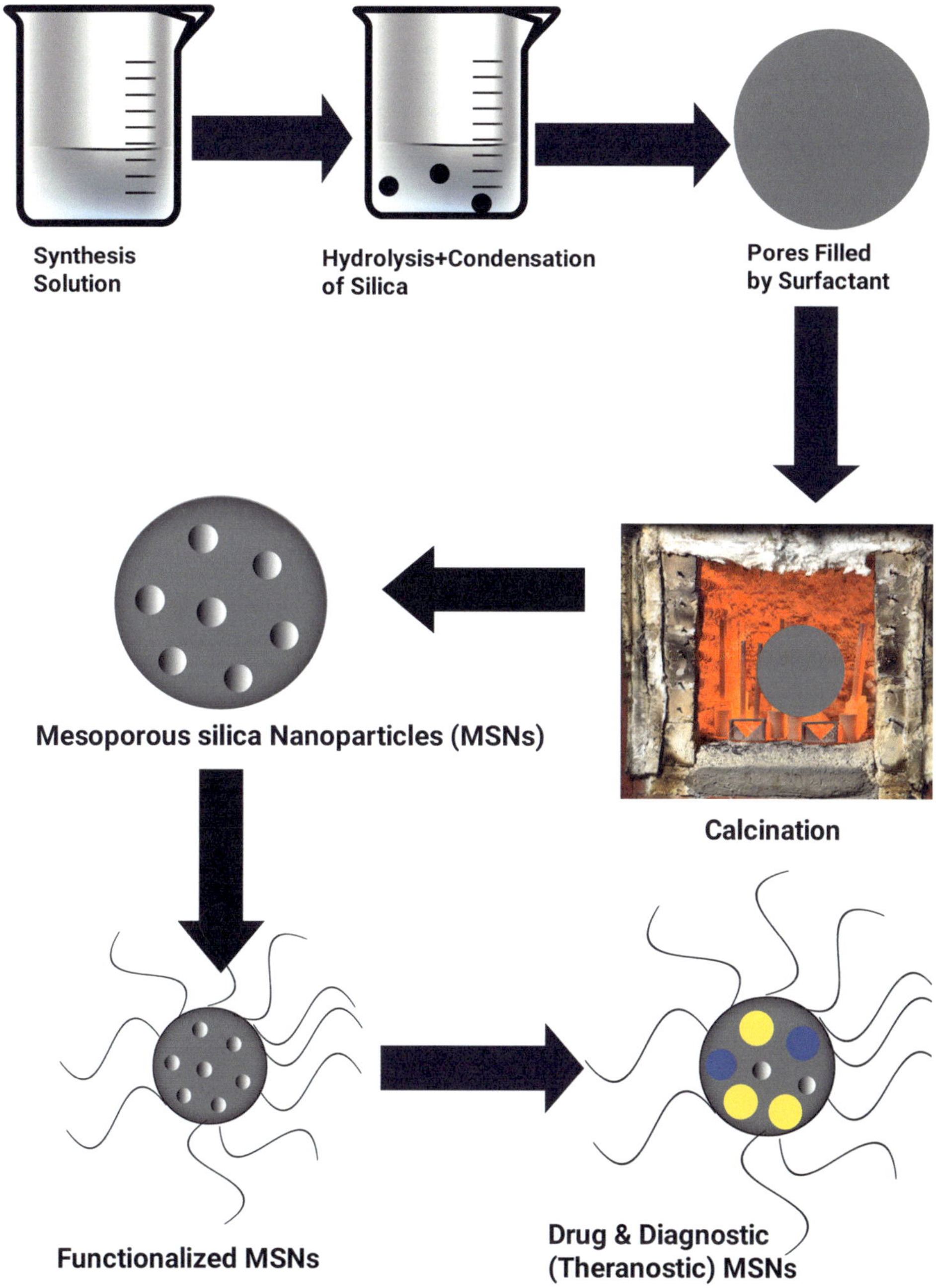

Figure 1.
Schematic representation of synthesis of MSNs.

intravenous administration by coupling with therapeutic agents [29]. Furthermore, the toxicity mitigation was attempted by conjugating the MSNPs with lipid matrices, which eventually demonstrated a substantial reduction in the toxicity of MCF-7 cells with regard to noncoated MSNPs after 48 h of incubation time [30]. The analysis of haemolysis also revealed relatively safe characteristics of the lipid-coated MSNPs over the uncoated ones. Recently, literature research on the production of PEG-coated

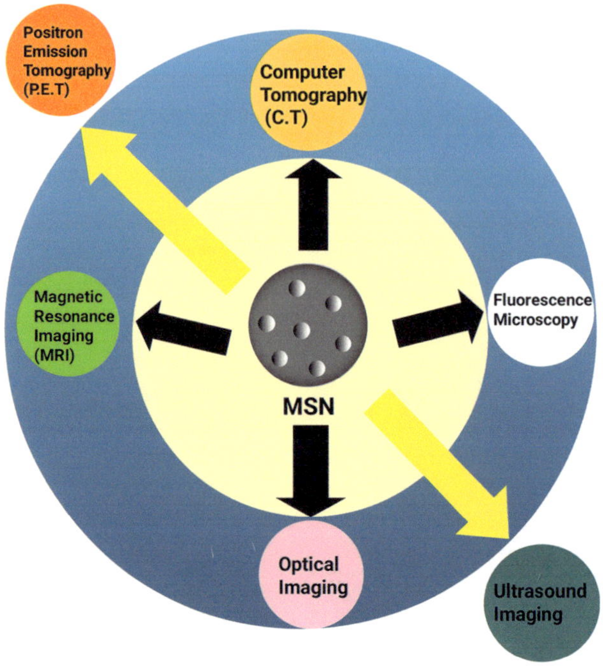

Figure 2.
Indicates different diagnostic techniques for cancer using MSNs.

Type	Internal structure	Pore size	Reference
MCM 41	2D Hexagonal	1.5–3.5	[21]
MCM 41	Hexagonal Structure with unidirectional pore structure	3.70	[22]
SBA 15	2D Hexagonal	6.0–10.0	[21]
SBA 15	2D Hexagonal	7.80	[22]
SBA 15	3D cubic cage like	4.0–9.0	[23]
MCM 48	3D cubic	2.5–3.0	[24]

Table 2.
Types & properties of MSNs.

organic-inorganic hybrid silica nano system (HMONs) reported substantially improved biodegradability and biocompatibility properties. The in vivo cytotoxicity assessment of the developed HMONs also did not disclose any significant pathophysiological improvements in the main organs (heart, liver, spleen, lung and kidney), which also verified in vivo biocompatibility of the PEG-conjugated HMONs [31].

6.2 Multidisciplinary nature of Mesoporous silica

Mesoporous Silica as Biosensor: The surface to volume ratio of NPs is very high, which enables ample functional ligands to be integrated and also allows multivalence on the surface of NP, which strengthens interactions with targets. MSN derivatives are often capped and gated in order to manipulate their applications in Controlled-release systems (CRS). In order to build different biosensors, various detection technologies were combined with the CRS [2, 32, 33].

Mesoporous Silica as Solubility Enhancer: The solubility enhancement mechanism of the mesoporous silica is clearly associated with the conversion of unstable crystalline form to stable amorphous form. Mesoporous silica has proved to be advantageous for poorly soluble drugs in increasing its solubility. MSNs have a high specific surface area, high pore volume and appropriate pore sizes in the molecular range, ordered pore structures and silanol groups on their surfaces that can interact with a variety of drug molecules. It also protects drug from external environment [34, 35].

Mesoporous Silica as wound healing aid: Mesoporous silica has found its application in this field as well. Nanoparticles have the ability to glue together the tissues by nano bridging effect. Nanobridging requires a particle size less than 100 nm while the clotting of blood depends on the porosity and the particle size of MSNs [36, 37].

7. Carrier and conjugate mediated DDS via MSN's

The main explanation behind the simple alteration of silica nanoparticles is silanol groups. With abundant and commercially available silane reagents, these groups can react. Then Silanes add other functional groups to the silica nanoparticles surface. The most commonly utilized silanes, along with different alkylsilane, PEG-silanes, have amine or sulfur groups at the end. Amine or thiol-ended groups give a simple linking chemistry with widely used molecules such as functionalized N-hydroxysuccinide (NHS), isothiocyanates, maleimides etc. [38, 39]. It is also possible to use each of these functional groups to tune the surface charge of the silica nanoparticles [40, 41]. Alkylsilanes are used for the treatment of hydrophobic surfaces and for increasing the echogenicity of silica nanoparticles. PEG-silanes graft PEG onto silica nanoparticles, increase the durability of the particles in biological fluids and extend the circulation period in vivo [42, 43]. Below **Table 3** presents the most commonly used silanes and their purposes for nanoparticle surface modification.

Methods Employed for Surface Functionalization of MSNPs.

Methods employed for surface functionalization of MSNPs are shown below

a. Co-Condensation

b. Multifunctionalization

c. Grafting

1. Co-condensation process (one-pot synthesis)

The direct condensation of organosilanes with a combination of silica precursors and surfactant templates is co-condensation. The process of co-condensation provides the probability of providing homogeneously dispersed organic groups without pore-blockage or shrinkage problems on the complete inner pore surfaces [56]. Also, the morphology of MSNPs can be regulated by the incorporation of various organosilanes. Researchers also observed that organosilanes with hydrophobic groups interact with surfactant hydrophobic tails, allowing the organic groups of organosilanes to be intercalated with the surfactant micelles [57, 58]. This leads to long cylindrical

Silanes	Functional Group	Application	Ref
(3-aminopropyl) trimethoxysil ane (APTMS)	-NH2	Reduced aggregation, Fluorescent labelling	[44, 45]
(3-aminopropyl) triethoxysilan e (APTES)	NH2	Surface charge modification, DNA binding and protection from enzymatic cleavage	[46]
(3-mercaptopropyl)-trimethox ysilane (MPTMS)	-SH	Conjugate with maleimides1, Thiol/disulfide exchange reactions to attach oligonucleotides, Surface charge modification	[47–49]
Polyethylene glycol-silane (PEG-silane)	-PEG	Increased circulation time, Reduced aggregation and increase particle dispersity in aqueous solution	[50]
Alkyl silane	Alkyl chain	Hydrophobic coating, Increase ultrasound contrast	[51, 52]
Carboxyethylsilanetriol	-COOH	Functionalize silica NPs and provide reactive sites for amine	[53]
3-trihydroxysilylpropyl methylphosphonate	-PO3	Functionalize silica NPs and provide reactive sites for amine	[54]
(3-isocyanatopropyl)-triethoxysilane	-NCO	Functionalize silica NPs and provide reactive sites for amine	[55]

Table 3.
Different functionalization of MSNs.

micelles being stabilized, and MSNPs are obtained in rod shapes. Hydrophilic organosilanes, on the contrary, do not interfere with surfactants and no further micelle stabilization exists, creating spherical particles with spontaneously directed pore structures. In binding with surfactant molecules, functional groups with a greater capacity to compete with silicate anions will be more likely to occur on MSNP surfaces than those weakly binding functional groups that are normally embedded in the silica frameworks and are thus unavailable [59].

2. Grafting method (Post-Synthesis Modification)

Grafting modifies a prefabricated inorganic mesoporous NP surface by adding functional groups to the material surface, typically after elimination of surfactants, and is thus a form of post-synthesis. The surface silanol groups (Si- OH) of MSNPs, typically present in high concentrations, serve as adequate anchoring points for organic functionalization in this process. Silylation is often achieved through surface functionalization of organic groups by grafting. The process of silylation takes place on free (≡Si—OH) and geminal silanol (=Si(OH)2) groups. Hydrogen-bonded silanol groups, however, form hydrophilic networks and functionalization is carried out to a small degree. Functionalization is conducted on the outer surface and at the opening of the pores of MSNPs in the grafting process. The drawback of grafting is the inhomogeneity in the coverage of surfaces because silanols are kinetically more accessible on the outside surface and at the opening of the mesopores than those located in the inner pore walls. Organosilane grafted MSNPs have better preserved pore structures as compared to co-condensed MSNPs and are more thermally stable. In most cases, due to the small amount of free surface silanol groups, the degree of functionalization by the grafting process is lower than that of the co-condensation method [59].

3. Multifunctionalization

It is beneficial to be able to combine more than one form of functional group with the MSNPs in order to create a more complex MSNP-based DDS. It is possible to co-condense two different organosilanes with silica precursors, but different silane hydrolysis rates will weaken the ordering of MSNPs and reduce the quantity of loading. In addition, the positions of the functional groups cannot be strictly controlled. Therefore, for the selective integration of functional groups into the external and internal surface of MSNPs, the multifunctionalization approach was developed using both cocondensation and grafting methods. The MSNPs are first synthesized using the cocondensation method in this step, and the free groups of silanols are then functionalized in a supercritical fluid medium using the grafting method. The surfactant is then extracted in this synthesis with the extraction of alcohol acid, resulting in the forming of the mesoporous structure [59].

8. Theranostic applications of MSN's

Nanoparticles serving as both diagnostic and therapeutic agents are theranostic and multimodal imageable nanoparticles. Theranostic nanoparticles are useful instruments for the detection and selection of patients followed by supportive care. The benefits of various imaging modalities are combined by multimodal nanoparticle contrast agents. The toxicity of nanoparticles that contain harmful components such as heavy metals can also be minimized by silica. Another useful technique for making multifunctional nanoparticles is doping functional elements such as lanthanide ions into silica. Gadolinium (Gd), for example, is a widely used MRI T1 contrast agent but it is toxic due to its concentration in tissues such as the liver, bone, and kidneys. Gadolinium-doped silica nanoparticles not only increase the contrast of the MRI but also decrease the toxicity of Gd (**Figure 3**) [60].

Rieter et al. attached a silylated Gd complex paramagnetic monolayer to a Luminescent [Ru(2,2′-bypyridine)3] Cl2 with reverse microemulsion core by a water-in - oil process. Due to the [Ru(2,2′-bypyridine)3] Cl2 centre and the Gd in the silica cap, this nanoparticle supplies fluorescent and MRI signals. Also, silica is conjugated with diethylenetriaminetetraacetate (DTTA), which generates seven binding sites for Gd^{3+} ions to reduce nanoparticles' toxicity due to Gd^{3+} core leaching. The nanoparticle is tiny enough (< 50 nm) to be endocytized by monocyte cells, which enables cells to be imaged multimodally in vitro. This nanoparticle is used by the investigators as target-specific contrast agents for optical and magnetic resonance imaging (MR) of rheumatoid arthritis in mice [61].

Photoacoustic (PA) imaging combining optical and ultrasound benefits have been developed to enhance diagnosis accuracy and sensitivity for early stage tumors, which offers the best resolution in deep tissue relative to some traditional imaging methods [62]. Thus, PA imaging, conveniently paired with ultrasound imaging, will greatly increase clinical diagnosis in the integrated method [63]. To this end, a conjugate of hyaluronate-silica nanoparticle (HA – SiNP) was synthesized by Lee and colleagues as a PA contrast agent: An MSNs-based liver targeting therapy. The PA amplitude in the liver after HA-SiNP conjugate injection was dramatically improved by 95.9 percent relative to standard liver over other PA contrast agents due to the powerful photoacoustic signal of SiNP in NIR windows, which offers more anatomical and functional information for HCC diagnosis [64].

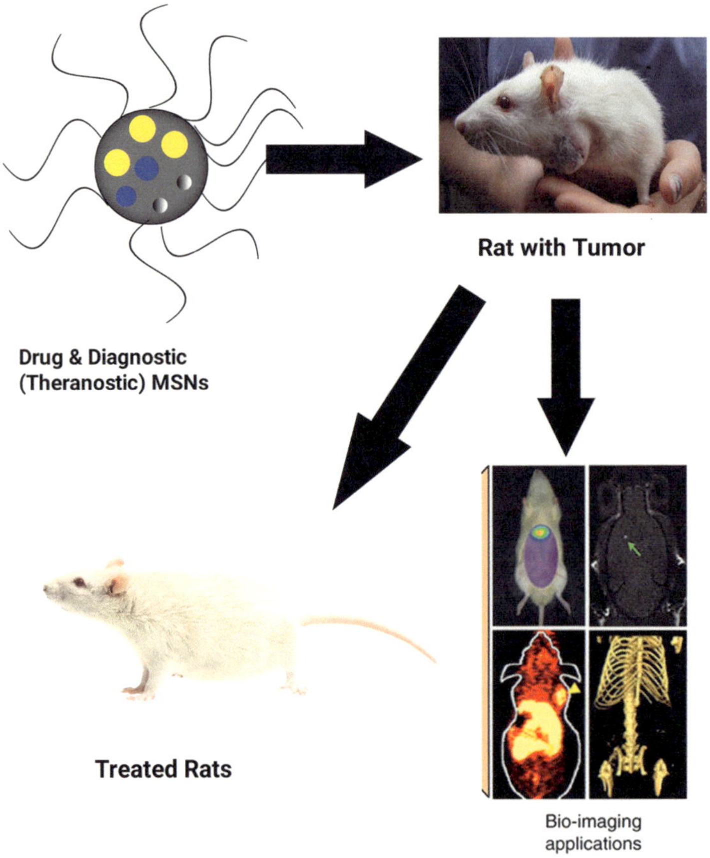

Figure 3.
Theranostic application of mesoporous silica.

As an activatable theranostic agent, Suk Ho Hong and associates developed an Indocyanine green-loaded hollow mesoporous silica nanoparticle. They became highly fluorescent once the nanoparticles reached the cancer cells through endocytosis. The study was carried out using cellular uptake quantitative analysis, in vitro cytotoxicity and in vitro phototoxicity research. The substance has shown significant potential for selective fluorescent NIR cancer [65]. Pegah Khosravian and Folic acid/methionine processed and tested, functionalizes mesoporous silica nanoparticles for docetaxel distribution. Usage of 3-aminopropyl triethoxy silane to achieve amine functionalisation. In vivo and ex vivo fluorescence imaging, In vivo application of nanoparticles, infrared and spectroscopy test MSNs, MTT assay, SEM, TEM. With small size distribution, the synthesized MSN-NH2 exhibited an average diameter of 49 nm. MSNs with a narrow size distribution, functionalized and DTX-loaded [66]. Hartono and colleagues 2016, prepared a system for curcumin bioavailability enhancement; which was intended for oral use. It possessed cubic shaped MSNs. It possessed better release profile and a higher solubility. Physical characterization was carried out by using TEM, XRD, FTIR, In-vitro release studies. Higher bioavailability of MSN-A-Cur and MSM-A-Cur was observed when compared to that of free curcumin. Pore size of 1.8 nm was observed in amine functionalized MCM-41 [67].

N. Lashgari and associates in 2016 demonstrated that as solid chemosensors and various advanced hybrid materials modified by fluorescence molecules have recently been prepared, the organic–inorganic hybrid nanomaterials have major advantages. In the other hand, mesoporous silica's homogeneous porosity and wide surface area make it a promising inorganic help [68].

Pande Vishal and colleagues 2018, mesoporous silica nanoparticles are produced as a targeted therapy medium that serves as a carrier for gemcitabine hydrochloride with fluorescein loaded onto nanoparticles for fluorescence microscopy tracing and imaging. As a target for pancreatic cancer cells, folic acid is conjugated with mesoporous silica nanoparticles [69]. Pande Vishal et al. 2020 produced a Targeted & Theranostic DDS using MSNs, fluorescein and magnetic nanoparticles. The therapeutic agent used in this system was gemcitabine hydrochloride. The folic acid functionalisation to the MSNs guided it to the cancer cells while the fluorescein and magnetic nanoparticles can be traced with the help of suitable technique and played the role of diagnostic agents in the system. The system showed excellent invitro anticancer activity and superior in vivo bioavailability was found in case of MSNs as compared to plain drug [70].

A flexible of mesoporous silica is engineered by Zang& colleagues in 2019 and worked on the basis of aqueous well-dispersed, including ion doping, surface alteration and pore adsorption. Thus, by endowing certain specific materials, a multifunctional theranostic nanoplatform is obtained. Gd ions are added to mesoporous silica (GM nanoparticles) in depth via a co-assembly process, which is used as the primary MRI carrier. In addition, the hyaluronic acid (HA) molecule surface graft leads to lymph system-targeted distribution (GMH nanoparticles). In addition, the development of Iopamidol (IGMH nanoparticles) and DOX (DGMH nanoparticles) functional molecules could integrate diagnosis and treatment with CT and sustained drug release. They present evidence that IGMH and DGMH nanoparticles are strongly active in vitro and in vivo for the lymphatic system, emphasizing CT and MR imaging of IGMH nanoparticles in the lymphatic system and chemotherapy and MR imaging of DGMH nanoparticles in lymphatic cancer [71]. Nihal Elbialy et al. 2019, Synthesized smart theranostic Platform of PEGylated mesoporous silica nanoparticles loaded-curcumin for the prevention and treatment of cancer. This Nanocarrier increased Bioavailability of Curcumin as well as provided a self-Fluorescent System for bioimaging of cancer [72].

9. Conclusions

In this review we have discussed different types of cancer & its therapies. We have specially emphasized on Mesoporous silica, its functionalisation and its use as Theranostic Medicine. Mesoporous silica with different diagnostic agents facilitated drug delivery to targeted site and at cellular level. Different diagnostic aids help its tracing. Various external stimuli may lead its path toward the target site or may be opted by the functionalisation done on the surface. While preclinical trials of MSNs have been successfully performed, there are currently no MSNs approved to be used in clinics. There are some crucial problems for MSNs that need to be resolved. First, the latest small animal models are not sufficient to test the delivery efficacy and long-term toxicity of nanoparticles in humans. Secondly, the production of MSNs on the laboratory scale cannot easily be replicated on the industrial scale of production for clinical use, especially in the case of complex modified MSNs. Third, there is no rigorous appraisal criteria that may confused the researchers to enhance the current MSNs. These problems when solved can lead to a potential formulation development based on MSNs for cancer Theranostic.

Acronyms and abbreviations

MSNs	Mesoporous silica Nanoparticles
GRAS	Generally recognized as safe
MCM	Mobil Crystalline Materials
SBA	Santa Barbara Amorphous
DDS	Drug Delivery Systems

Author details

Ajinkya Pote[1*], Vikas Ahirrao[2] and Vishal Pande[2]

1 Matoshri Institute of Pharmacy, Yeola, India

2 Rastriya Shikshan Mandal NN Sattha College of Pharmacy, Ahmednagar, India

*Address all correspondence to: ajinkyapote1996@gmail.com

References

[1] Sambi M, Bagheri L, Szewczuk MR. Current challenges in cancer immunotherapy: Multimodal approaches to improve efficacy and patient response rates. Journal of Oncology. 2019:1-12

[2] Pote A, Pande VV, Patel VP, Giri MA. Aniket Uttam Pund and Nitin Vijay Shelke, State of the art review on emerging applications of Mesoporous silica. The Open Nanomedicine and Nanotechnology Journal. 2020;**6**:12-20. DOI: 10.2174/2666150002006010012

[3] https://www.cancer.gov/about-cancer/treatment/types

[4] Lin Y-S, Haynes CL. Impacts of Mesoporous silica nanoparticle size, pore ordering, and pore integrity on hemolytic activity. Journal of the American Chemical Society. 2010;**132**(13):4834-4842

[5] CRA. Five Challenges to Improving Access to Cancer Treatments Market Access and Pricing in Emerging Markets. Boston: CRA; 2019

[6] Zugazagoitia J, Guedes C, Ponce S, Ferrer I, Molina-Pinelo S, Paz-Ares L. Current challenges in cancer treatment. Clinical Therapeutics. 2016;**38**(7): 1551-1566. DOI: 10.1016/j.clinthera.2016.03.026

[7] Humphrey LJ. Early detection of cancer. Seminars in Surgical Oncology. 1989;**5**(3):151-152

[8] Catena L. Targeted therapy. Tumori. 2010;**96**:861-865

[9] Dermime S. Carcinogenesis & Mutagenesis: Cancer diagnosis, treatment and therapy. J Carcinog Mutagen. 2013;**2013**:S14

[10] Guide WHO, Programmes E. Cancer Control - Diagnosis and Treatment. Geneva, Switzerland: WHO; 2008

[11] Roulston JE, Bartlett JMS. Molecular diagnosis of cancer. Mol Diagnosis Cancer. 2004;**97**:1-27

[12] Menasco D, Wang Q. Nanoparticles as drug delivery vehicles. Drug Deliv Princ Appl Second Ed. 2016;7(12):299-335

[13] De Jong WH, Borm PJA. Drug delivery and nanoparticles: Applications and hazards. International Journal of Nanomedicine. 2008;**3**(2):133-149

[14] Asefa T, Tao Z. Biocompatibility of mesoporous silica nanoparticles. Chemical Research in Toxicology. 2012;**25**(11):2265-2284

[15] Wilczewska AZ, Niemirowicz K, Markiewicz KH, Car H. Nanoparticles as drugdelivery systems. Pharmacol Reports. 2012;**64**(5):1020-1037. DOI: 10.1016/S1734-1140(12)70901-5

[16] Rizvi SAA, Saleh AM. Applications of nanoparticle systems in drug delivery technology. Saudi Pharm J [Internet]. 2018;**26**(1):64-70. DOI: 10.1016/j.jsps.2017.10.012

[17] LexInnova. Nanoparticles smart drug delivery system for cancer. LexInnova. 2013;**14**:1-43

[18] Mirjalili F, Soltani M, Chen P. Nanotechnology in drug delivery systems. Int J Drug Deliv. 2012;**4**(3):1-14

[19] Patil-sen Y. Nanoparticles: Smart drug delivery systems. Curr Trends Biomedical Eng & Biosci. 2018;**11**(3):21-23

[20] Kwon S, Singh RK, Perez RA, Abou Neel EA, Kim HW, Chrzanowski W. Silica-based mesoporous nanoparticles for controlled drug delivery. J Tissue Eng. 2013;**4**:1-18

[21] Vivero-Escoto JL, Luis J. Surface functionalized mesoporous silica nanoparticles for intracellular drug delivery. Dissertation Abstracts International. 2009;**71**:621-638

[22] Selvam P, Bhatia SK, Sonwane CG. Recent advances in processing and characterization of periodic mesoporous MCM-41 silicate molecular sieves. Industrial and Engineering Chemistry Research. 2001;**40**:3237-3261

[23] Gary-Bobo M, Hocine O, Brevet D, Maynadier M, Raehm L, Richeter S, et al. Cancer therapy improvement with mesoporous silica nanoparticles combining targeting, drug delivery and PDT. International Journal of Pharmaceutics. 2012;**423**:509-515

[24] Yiu HH, Wright PA. Enzymes supported on ordered mesoporous solids: A special case of an inorganic-organic hybrid. Materials Chemistry. 2005;**15**:3690-3700

[25] Tourne-Peteilh C, Begu S, Lerner DA, Galarneau A, Lafont U, Devoisselle JM. Sol-gel one-pot synthesis in soft conditions of mesoporous silica materials ready for drug delivery system. J Solgel Sci Technol. 2012;**61**:455-462

[26] Liong M, Lu J, Kovochich M, Xia T, Ruehm SG, Nel AE, et al. Multifunctional inorganic nanoparticles for imaging, targeting, and drug delivery. ACS Nano. 2008;**2**(5):889-896

[27] Bollu VS, Barui AK, Mondal SK, Prashar S, Fajardo M, Briones D, et al. Curcumin-loaded silica-based mesoporous materials: Synthesis, characterization and cytotoxic properties against cancer cells. Materials Science and Engineering. 2016;**63**:393-410

[28] Wang L-S, Wu L-C, Lu S-Y, Chang L-L, Teng IT, Yang C-M, et al. Biofunctionalized phospholipid-capped Mesoporous silica Nanoshuttles for targeted drug delivery: Improved water Suspensibility and decreased nonspecific protein binding. ACS Nano. 2010;**4**(8):4371-4379

[29] Han N, Wang Y, Bai J, Liu J, Wang Y, Gao Y, et al. Facile synthesis of the lipid bilayer coated mesoporous silica nanocomposites and their application in drug delivery. Microporous and Mesoporous Materials. 2016;**219**:209-218. DOI: 10.1016/j.micromeso.2015.08.006

[30] Huang P, Chen Y, Lin H, Yu L, Zhang L, Wang L, et al. Molecularly organic/inorganic hybrid hollow mesoporous organosilica nanocapsules with tumor-specific biodegradability and enhanced chemotherapeutic functionality. Biomaterials. 2017;**125**:23-37. DOI: 10.1016/j.biomaterials.2017.02.018

[31] Bertrand N, Wu J, Xu X, Kamaly N, Farokhzad OC. Cancer nanotechnology: The impact of passive and active targeting in the era of modern cancer biology. Advanced Drug Delivery Reviews. 2014;**66**:2-25

[32] Chen Z, Tan Y, Xu K, et al. Stimulus-response mesoporous silica nanoparticle-based chemiluminescence biosensor for cocaine determination. Biosensors & Bioelectronics. 2016;**75**:8-14. DOI: 10.1016/j.bios.2015.08.006

[33] Zhu CL, Lu CH, Song XY, Yang HH, Wang XR. Bioresponsive controlled release using mesoporous silica nanoparticles capped with aptamer-based molecular gate. Journal

of the American Chemical Society. 2011;**133**(5):1278-1281. DOI: 10.1021/ja110094g

[34] Laitinen R, Löbmann K, Strachan CJ, Grohganz H, Rades T. Emerging trends in the stabilization of amorphous drugs. International Journal of Pharmaceutics. 2013;**453**(1):65-79. DOI: 10.1016/j.ijpharm.2012.04.066

[35] Hartono SB, Hadisoewignyo L, Yang Y, Meka AK, Antaresti YC. Amine functionalized cubic mesoporous silica nanoparticles as an oral delivery system for curcumin bioavailability enhancement. Nanotechnology. 2016;**27**(50):505605. DOI: 10.1088/0957-4484/27/50/505605

[36] Lu MM, Bai J, Shao D, et al. Antibacterial and biodegradable tissue nano-adhesives for rapid wound closure. International Journal of Nanomedicine. 2018;**13**:5849-5863

[37] Kim JH, Kim H, Choi Y, Lee DS, Kim J, Yi GR. Colloidal mesoporous silica nanoparticles as strong adhesives for hydrogels and biological tissues. ACS Applied Materials & Interfaces. 2017;**9**(37):31469-31477. DOI: 10.1021/acsami.7b09083

[38] Tsai CP, Chen CY, Hung Y, Chang FH, Mou CY. Monoclonal antibody-functionalized mesoporous silica nanoparticles (MSN) for selective targeting breast cancer cells. Journal of Materials Chemistry. 2009;**19**(32):5737-5743

[39] Peng JF, He XX, Wang KM, Tan WH, Wang Y, Liu Y. Nucleic acid conjugated Nanomaterials for enhanced molecular recognition. Analytical and Bioanalytical Chemistry. 2007;**388**(3):645-654

[40] Wang Y, Sun Y, Wang J, Yang Y, Li Y, Yuan Y, et al. CO2 Electroreduction at low Overpotential on oxide-derived Cu/carbons fabricated from metal organic framework. ACS Applied Materials & Interfaces. 2016;**8**(27):17166-17175

[41] Wang JX, Chen F, Arconada-Alvarez SJ, Hartanto J, Yap LP, Park R, et al. Multifunctional nanomedicine with silica: Role of silica in nanoparticles for theranostic, imaging, and drug monitoring. Nano Letters. 2016;**16**(10):6265-6271

[42] HeQ ZZ, Gao F, Li Y, Shi J. In vivo biodistribution and urinary excretion of mesoporous silica nanoparticles: Effects of particle size and PEGylation. Small. 2011;**7**(2):271-280

[43] Cauda V, Argyo C, Bein T. Impact of different PEGylation patterns on the long-term bio-stability of colloidal mesoporous silicananoparticles. Journal of Materials Chemistry. 2010;**20**(39):8693-8699

[44] Bagwe RP, Hilliard LR, Tan WL. Surface modification of silica nanoparticles to reduce aggregation and nonspecific binding. Langmuir. 2006;**22**(9):4357-4362

[45] Peng JF, He XX, Wang KM, Tan WH, Wang Y, Liu Y. Nucleic acid conjugated Nanomaterials for enhanced molecular recognition. Analytical and Bioanalytical Chemistry. 2007;**388**(3):645-654

[46] Wang Y, Sun Y, Wang J, Yang Y, Li Y, Yuan Y, et al. CO2 Electroreduction at low Overpotential on oxide-derived Cu/carbons fabricated from metal organic framework. ACS Applied Materials & Interfaces. 2016;**8**(27):17166-17175

[47] Tsai CP, Chen CY, Hung Y, Chang FH, Mou CY. Monoclonal antibody-functionalized mesoporous silica nanoparticles (MSN) for selective targeting breast cancer

cells. Journal of Materials Chemistry. 2009;**19**(32):5737-5743

[48] Tan WH, Wang KM, He XX, Zhao XJ, Drake T, Wang L, et al. Bionanotechnology based on silica nanoparticles. Medicinal Research Reviews. 2004;**24**(5):621-638

[49] Shaffer TM, Harmsen S, Khwaja E, Kircher MF, Drain CM, Grimm. Stable adiolabeling of sulfur-functionalized silica nanoparticles with Copper-64. J. Nano Letters. 2016;**16**(9):5601-5604

[50] Van Vlerken LE, Vyas TK, Amiji MM. Poly(ethylene glycol)-modified nanocarriers for tumor-targeted and intracellular delivery. Pharmaceutical Research. 2007;**24**(8):1405-1414

[51] Zhang X, Shi F, Niu J, Jiang YG, Wang ZQ. Superhydrophobic surfaces: From structural control to functional application. Journal of Materials Chemistry. 2008;**18**(6):621-633

[52] Jin QF, Lin CY, Kang ST, Chang YC, Zheng HR, Yang CM, et al. Multifunctional nanomedicine with silica: Role of silica in nanoparticles for theranostic, imaging, and drug monitoring. Ultrasonics Sonochemistry. 2017;**36**:262-269

[53] Zhang P, Kong J. Talanta. 2015;**134**(SupplementC):501-507

[54] Popat A, Liu J, Lu GQ, Qiao SZ. A pH-responsive drug delivery system based on chitosan coated mesoporous silica nanoparticles. Journal of Materials Chemistry. 2012;**22**(22):11173-11178

[55] Agostini A, Mondragón L, Coll C, Aznar E, Marcos MD, Martínez-Máñez R, et al. Temperature-controlled release by changes in the secondary structure of peptides anchored onto mesoporous silica supports. Chemistry Open. 2012;**1**(1):17-20

[56] Fabiola P. Mesoporous Silica Nanoparticles as Drug Delivery Systems. Division of Soft Chemistry Matter, Leiden Institute of Chemistry (LIC), Faculty of Science. The Netherlands: Leiden University; 2012

[57] Huang Y. Functionalization of Mesoporous Silica Nanoparticles and their Applications in Organo-, Metallic and Organometallic Catalysis (Dissertation). Iowa: Iowa State University; 2009

[58] Sun X. Mesoporoussilica Nanoparticlesfor Applicationsin Drug Delivery and Catalysis (Dissertation). Linköping: Linköping University; 2012

[59] Pednekar PP, Godiyal SC, Jadhav KR, Kadam VJ. Mesoporous silica nanoparticles: A promising multifunctional drug delivery system. Nanostructures for Cancer Therapy. 2017:593-621

[60] Rogosnitzky M, Branch S. Gadolinium-based contrast agent toxicity: A review of known and proposed mechanisms. Biometals. 2016;**29**:365-376

[61] Rieter WJ, Kim JS, Taylor KM, An H, Lin W, Tarrant T, et al. Hybrid silica nanoparticles for multimodal imaging. Angewandte Chemie. 2007;**119**(20):3754-3756

[62] Liu Y, Bhattarai P, Dai Z, Chen X. Photothermal therapy and photoacoustic imaging via nanotheranostics in fighting cancer. Chemical Society Reviews. 2019;**48**:2053-2108

[63] Kim J, Park S, Jung Y, Chang S, Park J, Zhang Y. Programmable real-time clinical photoacoustic and ultrasound

imaging system. Scientific Reports. 2016;**6**:35137

[64] Lee D, Beack S, Yoo J, Kim SK, Lee C, Kwon W. In vivo photoacoustic imaging of livers using biodegradable hyaluronic acid-conjugated silica nanoparticles. Advanced Functional Materials. 2018;**28**:1800941

[65] Hong SH, Kim H, Choi Y. Indocyanine green-loaded hollow Mesoporous silica nanoparticles as An Activatable Theranostic agent. Nanotechnol. 2017;**28**:1-8

[66] Khosravian P, Ardestani MS, Khoobi M, Ostad EN, Dorkoosh FA. Mesoporous silica nanoparticles functionalized with folic acid/ methionine for active targeted delivery of Docetaxel. Oncotargets and Therapy. 2016;**9**:7315-7330

[67] Hartono SB, Hadisoewignyo L, Yang Y, Meka AK, Antaresti Yu C. Amine functionalized cubic mesoporous silica nanoparticles as an oral delivery system for curcumin bioavailability enhancement. Nanotechnology. 2016;**22**(50):505605

[68] Lashgari N, Badiei A, Mohammadi ZG. Modification of mesoporous silica SBA-15 with different organic molecules to gain chemical sensors: A review. Nanochemistry Res. 2016;**1**(1):127-141

[69] Pande VV, Borawake DD, Halnor VV. Fabrication and characterization of gemcitabine hydrochloride loaded Mesoporous silica nanoparticles as Theranostics platform for pancreatic cancer. Materials and Technologies. 2018;**33**(13):815-824. DOI: 10.1080/10667857.2018.1512782

[70] Pande VV, Khedkar PV, Giri MA, Pote AK, Polshettiwar SA. Fabrication and characterisation of gemcitabine hydrochloride loaded magnetically responsive mesoporous silica nanocomposites as smart hybrid theranostic platform for treatment of pancreatic cancer. Materials Technology. 2020;**36**:145-152

[71] Zhang Y, Cheng J, Li N, Wang R, Huang G, Zhu J, et al. A versatile theranostic nanoplatform based on mesoporous silica. Materials Science and Engineering. 2019;**98**:560-571

[72] Elbialy NS, Aboushoushah SF, Sofi BF, Noorwali A. Multifunctional curcumin-loaded mesoporous silica nanoparticles for cancer chemoprevention and therapy. Microporous and Mesoporous Materials. 2019;**291**:109540. DOI: 10.1016/j. micromeso.2019.06.002